My Quiet War

How a Leader, a Family, and a Miracle Donor Gave

Me a Second Life

By Daniel O'Connell, EdD

Copyright Page

Publisher:

DocLogical Press

A Division of **DocLogical, LLC**

Avon, Connecticut, USA

www.doclogical.com

ISBN (Paperback): 979-8-9940993-0-8

Library of Congress Control Number: 2025927727

Cover Design: DocLogical Press Studio

Interior Design & Layout: DocLogical Press

December 2025

Printed in the United States of America

Dedication

To my donor, my family, and everyone still waiting for their miracle.
May this book bring to the journey, strength to the weary, and hope to every soul
still fighting for one more day.

Mission Statement / Social Impact Note

DocLogical, LLC proudly donates 2% of all sales to kidney health and veteran causes, including the National Kidney Foundation, PKD Foundation, and Wounded Warrior Project.

Foreword - A Medical Reflection on Resilience

By Sue Chang, MD - (Nephrologist) – Metabolism Associates

When I first met Daniel O'Connell, I saw a man defined not by illness, but by an unrelenting drive to live with purpose. His journey through Polycystic Kidney Disease (PKD) and Chronic Kidney Disease (CKD) was not simply about surviving a diagnosis; it was about transforming adversity into meaning, science into service, and recovery into leadership.

Over nearly two decades, Daniel faced what most would call insurmountable: the steady decline of kidney function, countless labs and procedures, and the uncertainty of transplant candidacy. Yet, throughout it all, he continued to teach, mentor, and lead, guiding students, executives, and patients alike with the same steadiness that once guided his Navy missions.

This book, *My Quiet War, How a Leader, a Family, and a Miracle Donor Gave Me a Second Life,* is more than a memoir. It's a blueprint for hope. Within these pages, Daniel gives voice to the silent battles faced by millions living with kidney disease, and he does so with authenticity, intelligence, and compassion.

For patients, this is a guide.
For caregivers, this is understanding.
For clinicians, this is a perspective.

For all of us, this is proof that resilience is not born in comfort but forged in challenge. 'But they that wait upon the Lord shall renew their strength; they shall mount up with wings as eagles; they shall run, and not be weary; and they shall walk, and not faint.' Isaiah 40:31.

Sue Chang, MD
Metabolism Associates, New Haven, CT

Foreword – A Gift of Life

By Ryan Long - (Donor)

Faith. Family. Purpose. Honor. These are pillars that have long resonated with me, compass points to help guide me through life's challenges, large and small. Every so often, the universe presents us with quiet moments where choices not only test our values but gently re-orient the compass of our lives.

One such moment arrived when I learned that Dan, a man whose life had been marked by extraordinary service, was facing the greatest battle of his life.

Long before becoming a kidney donor was something I had ever imagined, Dan and I met when we both started working at Gotham Greens in Brooklyn, NY, on a summer day in July 2019. In fact, we started on the exact same day, nearly seven years ago. I remember recognizing early on there was something different about Dan, a steadiness, a presence shaped by a depth of experience few people come to know.

Years later, when I learned of Dan's illness - Polycystic Kidney Disease, or PKD - I felt something I didn't expect: anger. How could someone who had given so much of his life to others suddenly find himself facing a silent, genetic disease that he did nothing to deserve?

It seemed to violate a deeper code - that someone who had carried others through danger was now being asked to carry this burden by himself.

I'd known Dan as a man of high caliber, principle, faith, and service. Someone who had forged an early career as a Navy Corpsman - trained to run toward challenge, not away from it. Someone who had endured the dust, danger, and chaos of incoming fire at night and combat zone landings in Baghdad, as simply part of the job. A man who, after serving in the Navy, reinvented himself as a civilian pilot, then again as a teacher, technologist, mentor, and leader. Dan's life seemed a long arc of service, reinvention, and purpose.

At the time I considered donating, I was physically strong - fresh off a triathlon - but spiritually restless. I attended Mass regularly but felt drawn toward a more active expression of service. In faith terms, I had always admired St. Francis of Assisi, who taught that faith can be best expressed not in sentiment but in action. Perhaps it was a quiet foreshadowing of the confirmation name I chose at age eleven - Francis -of a future call to service.

And what clearer way to live one's faith than to give the gift of life?

Saying yes to serve as a kidney donor for Dan felt less like a sacrifice and more like alignment, the moment where what I believed met what I was meant to do. When you admire someone's character, someone's courage, someone's relentless commitment to others, the decision to help is not dramatic. It simply feels right.

Saint Francis wrote: "Happy is the servant who does not remain content with the reward of words." Perhaps sometimes faith can be most appropriately expressed through action. Humanity expressed through sacrifice. A commitment to something greater than ourselves is most authentic when it comes at a cost.

The story in these pages is Dan's. But I suppose in some sense, perhaps they're also a call to seek purpose in something greater than ourselves. Dan's battle did not begin alone; it continued from the moment a simple "yes" set a mission into motion. And as I read his words, I see a warrior who never surrendered, a pilot who refused grounding to define him, a leader who kept leading under fire, and a teacher who kept teaching even when the body faltered.

The kidney I gifted to Dan allowed him to continue the life of service he had been living for so long, service to students, colleagues, veterans, family, and now to every reader inspired by his resilience. His journey fulfills what every donor hopes for: that the gift will multiply meaning, purpose, and light in someone who carries it forward.

If warrior spirituality is real, Dan embodies it.

May this memoir honor not only those who fight for life, but also those who are blessed to help carry others forward.

-Ryan Long

Foreword – Brotherhood Beyond the Uniform

By Jason Burke, CAPT, USN (Ret.) - (Colleague)

I met Dan O'Connell in 2013, shortly after I was hired at Quinnipiac University in Hamden, Connecticut. We quickly became friends that stemmed from our service in the U.S. Navy and bonded by the lack of former military in higher education. Occasionally, we'd find time to catch up after work. During one of these happy hours, Dan confided to me that he was battling a life-threatening kidney disease and would need a transplant. What struck me then, and still today, was Dan's operational tempo. He's a CIO, working towards his doctoral degree, teaching, consulting, and writing. I found it hard to believe that he could be sick when he appeared to be in great health and emotional spirit.

The evening before his transplant surgery, Dan texted me that he was grateful to have me as a friend and colleague. I read between the lines that he was saying thank you and goodbye if this surgery was not successful. As a 'glass half full' guy, I felt Dan was going to be fine, and perhaps he was being a bit dramatic. However, I should know that Dan is never overdramatic, and after reading *My Quiet War*, I realize now how close he was to oblivion.

In war, to be victorious requires a sound strategy. A strategy or end state that stems from a thoughtful tactical and operational focus that is deliberate and adaptable. There's no difference with the approach to personal battles, and the pages that follow show how Dan's early nurture, along with his Navy training, provides a systematic approach of checklists, measurements, inquiries, and adaptation to setbacks that are key to survival. He also relies on faith and family, that direct mental and emotional focus with his day-to-day life, coinciding with his looming kidney failure. His story is one of resilience, balance, and mission focus. I believe he beat death for one reason: so that you might be encouraged by how he survived.

Jason Burke
CAPT, USN (Ret.)

Preface

In 2007, my life changed with three simple words: "You have PKD."

At the time, I didn't fully grasp what that meant. I had spent years in technology, aviation, and education, leading teams, teaching students, and helping others achieve clarity through data and systems. Suddenly, I was facing a system inside my own body that I couldn't repair, optimize, or replace.

Over the years that followed, I learned that chronic kidney disease isn't just a medical condition; it's a life condition. It reshapes how you think, plan, eat, travel, and even dream. It forces you to measure time not by milestones, but by lab results. Yet, within those numbers and challenges, I discovered something more profound: the extraordinary human capacity for resilience.

This book was born from that discovery.

I wrote My Quiet War to share my journey, not as a hero's story, but as a human one. I wanted to offer insight, hope, and practical guidance for anyone living with kidney disease, supporting a loved one through it, or simply trying to make sense of life's unexpected turns. My goal is to demystify what PKD and CKD truly mean, while highlighting the courage, science, and compassion that make survival and thriving possible.

For patients, I hope these pages provide reassurance that you are not alone.

For caregivers and families, I hope they illuminate what your loved ones experience but may never say aloud.

And for healthcare professionals, I hope this book serves as a reminder that beyond every diagnosis is a person striving to live, contribute, and inspire.

Today, more than a year after my kidney transplant, I live with renewed strength, gratitude, and purpose. My journey was never just about kidneys; it was about rediscovering what it means to be alive, connected, and purposeful.

If even one reader finds clarity, comfort, or courage in these pages, then this book will have fulfilled its mission.

Daniel O'Connell, EdD

Acknowledgments

No journey of healing is ever traveled alone. Though this book carries my name, it stands on the shoulders of countless people whose compassion, skill, and faith made every step possible.

To my family and friends, thank you for your love, patience, and constant belief that better days were ahead. You carried me through the most challenging moments and celebrated every small victory as if it were your own. Your strength became my anchor.

To my donor and his family, whose selfless act of generosity gave me a second chance at life, there are no words large enough to contain my gratitude. I live every day with a profound awareness of that gift and the responsibility it carries.

To my medical team, the extraordinary physicians, surgeons, nurses, coordinators, and specialists who walked beside me through the years of PKD, CKD, and ultimately transplantation, thank you for your unwavering dedication. You are the true engineers of hope. A special thanks to my nephrology and transplant teams at Yale New Haven Health, whose expertise and empathy turned science into salvation.

To my friends and colleagues, who never let illness define me or limit my purpose. Whether in data, AI, education, or leadership, your encouragement kept me connected to the world beyond the hospital walls. You reminded me that I still had something to teach, something to build, and something to give.

To my students, who continually inspired me with their curiosity and determination. Teaching while managing a chronic illness taught me more about perspective and gratitude than any classroom ever could.

To my Navy brothers and sisters, thank you for the lessons in discipline, teamwork, and endurance that became the foundation of my recovery. The same mindset that kept me aloft in the cockpit helped me navigate the storms of illness with resolve.

And finally, to everyone living with PKD, CKD, or waiting for a transplant, this book is for you. You are stronger than you know. May these pages remind you that life after diagnosis is not an ending, but the beginning of a new and extraordinary chapter.

With deep gratitude and renewed life,
Dr. Daniel O'Connell EdD
Avon, Connecticut
November 2025

Disclaimer

This book reflects my personal experience and should not be interpreted as medical advice.

Always consult qualified medical professionals regarding your own health decisions.

Table of Contents

Prologue

Before my kidneys failed, before the lab results, before the word *transplant* ever entered a room with my name attached to it, there was a boy formed by places, people, and principles that built the architecture of my resilience long before I ever needed it.

I was conceived in New York City, but I came into the world a few thousand miles south, on the island of Puerto Rico, a U.S. territory that at the time felt like a distant outpost of my father's work. He was a federal agent stationed there, and my earliest days were marked by sun, humidity, and the rhythm of an island I was too young to remember but somehow still feel in my bones.

At three years old, we came back to New York, settling in Staten Island, just close enough to Manhattan to feel its pull, but far enough away to have a world of its own. That borough became the backdrop of my childhood: neighborhood streets, tight-knit families, the smell of the ocean on certain days, and the particular blend of grit and humor that only New Yorkers truly understand.

Heritage mattered in our home. My father was Irish; his parents were born on the other side of the Atlantic, which meant I entered this world not only as an American but also an Irish citizen. My mother brought Italian and Spanish roots into the mix, creating a culture defined by humor, faith, warmth, intensity, and more than a few spirited discussions around the dinner table. It was loud, loving, imperfect, and real. I didn't know it then, but identity would become one of my greatest stabilizers later in life.

What my parents gave me was more than culture; it was a framework. Faith wasn't optional; it was oxygen. Service wasn't abstract; it was modeled daily. Discipline wasn't punishment; it was preparation. That foundation became the bedrock for everything that followed.

In 1991, right after high school, I joined the United States Navy as a Hospital Corpsman. I didn't know it then, but the Navy would become the crucible that forged my sense of duty, resilience, and mental discipline. It taught me how to compartmentalize under pressure, how to act when emotion wanted to freeze me, and how to lead even when uncertainty was the only certainty. Medicine, trauma, warfare, responsibility, those were not academic concepts; they were daily realities.

Ironically, what the Navy gave me in discipline, life took back in vision. In 1994, when I was allowed to fly for the Navy, during undergraduate flight training, a routine flight physical examination revealed my left eye was 20/200. In that era, that grounding was absolute. The dream of military aviation evaporated in minutes.

But grounded isn't the same as defeated.

I returned to Connecticut, where my parents had retired, and I kept flying anyway. Helicopters, gliders, airplanes, if it could get off the ground, I wanted my hands on the controls. Aviation became more than a skill; it became a metaphor for everything that came later. When the system told me "no", I found another way. When one path closed, I carved a new one. That pattern, adapt, adjust, ascend, became the mental choreography of my life.

Then, in 1997, my father passed unexpectedly. Five years later, my mother followed him. Those losses carved a permanent space inside me, but they also reshaped my understanding of time, mortality, and responsibility. You learn quickly, when both of your parents are gone before you turn thirty, that life is not measured in guarantees. It's measured in choices.

Those years also pushed me deeper into work, education, leadership, and service. I built a career, taught at universities, started consulting, and continued building a life rooted in faith and purpose. From the outside, it may have looked like momentum, achievement, or ambition. But in truth, it was preparation, a long runway leading toward a storm I had no idea was gathering.

Because everything changed in 2007.

One sentence, one scan, one consultation I never saw coming.

I didn't realize it then, but every moment of my early life, Navy discipline, aviation training, faith, loss, leadership, and the multicultural, service-driven home I was raised in, had been equipping me for the battle ahead. PKD didn't arrive in an empty landscape; it arrived in a mind already trained for adversity.

The resilience that carried me through the darkest moments of kidney failure wasn't created suddenly. It was inherited, refined, tested, and lived long before the diagnosis.

And so the story of my transplant doesn't begin with a lab number.

It begins here, in the places and people who built the man I had to become long before I knew why.

I

The Diagnosis

Chapter 1

When the World Changes

The year was 2007. The first hints of spring were finally visible after another long Connecticut winter, thin sunlight spilling over the still-bare trees, the kind of morning that makes you believe life is just beginning again. I was thirty-four, a husband, a father of three small children, and a consulting manager at Oracle Corporation. My life was all movement: airports, client sites, conference rooms, hotels. I traveled across the United States, Canada, and Europe, living out of a suitcase more than I lived out of drawers at home.

Sunday nights were flights; Friday nights were reunions. I would drop my bag by the door, scoop up whichever child ran toward me first, and try to squeeze a week's worth of family into forty-eight hours before the next flight. I told myself this was success, that motion equaled meaning. I worked hard, played hard, stayed fit, and believed I could outpace anything life threw at me.

When I wasn't working, I could usually be found at the Irish American Home in Glastonbury, surrounded by friends, a pint of Guinness in hand, sometimes playing Gaelic football until my knees gave out. Or at the gym, chasing the same sense of control I carried from my Navy days, discipline, routine, focus. Occasionally, I'd head to the range, line up my sights, and burn off the tension that travel and responsibility created. Those routines were my armor: sweat, laughter, noise, and momentum.

On the surface, everything looked solid. Inside, though, I was a complex equation of exhaustion and purpose. I still carried the quiet echoes of service-related trauma, the kind that doesn't announce itself but sits in the corners of your mind. I had lost my father a decade earlier, my mother five years after that. Somewhere between grief and duty, I learned to keep my head down and keep moving. Spiritually, I prayed often but never felt I deserved to be heard. I believed in God, but I thought I had disappointed Him more times than I could count.

That spring, I thought I was indestructible.

At that time, I was living life at full throttle. I had been a licensed pilot since 1994, flying both airplanes and helicopters, and I found freedom in the sky that few experiences could match. I was also a certified SCUBA diver and, for a time, a skydiver, always chasing the next horizon. But as the years passed, I began to slow some of those pursuits. I hadn't skydived since 1999, and by 2007, without even realizing it, I had already taken my last flight at the controls. The uncertainty of what my body might do next, the subtle fatigue, the awareness that something wasn't quite right, began to ground me in ways I didn't yet understand. Even then, I couldn't have imagined how much life was about to change.

The Fall (2005)

It really began in 2005, though I didn't recognize it then, a cool September Saturday around 7 a.m. I had just woken up and was heading downstairs with my daughter, who was four at the time. She wanted to go first, her small hand brushing the banister as she carefully took each step. I followed a few steps behind, half-awake, thinking about the day ahead. Then, without warning, the world went black.

There was no dizziness, no pain, just an instant void. One second, I was standing; the next, I was falling. I remember nothing of the impact, only the sound of voices when I opened my eyes again. I was at the bottom of the stairs, my daughter crying somewhere above me, and paramedics asking questions that floated through the haze: my name, what happened, could I move?

Training took over. Somewhere deep inside, the Navy corpsman in me, the medic I had once been, started triaging my own injuries, though my body wouldn't obey. One of the medics placed a hand on my shoulder and said, "Buddy, we've got this."

I was taken by ambulance to Yale–New Haven Hospital. Scans and MRIs followed. The doctors said I had blacked out completely, but, by some stroke of luck, had no fractures, just a concussion and a bruised arm that ached for weeks.

At the time, we all wrote it off as a fluke, a fainting episode. But in hindsight, that fall was the first signal that something deeper was wrong, the prologue to the years of tests and diagnoses that would follow.

The Pain

The first sign that something was wrong came out of nowhere. A sharp, searing pain bloomed just under my ribcage, so sudden it stole my breath. At first, I thought it was food poisoning or muscle strain from a workout. But when it returned, deeper, hotter, I knew it wasn't ordinary. Over the next few days, the pain grew unbearable. I remember sitting in an airport lounge, hunched over my briefcase, pretending everything was fine. It wasn't.

Within a week, I was in my doctor's office describing the sensation as if someone were stabbing me from the inside. He ordered an ultrasound, suspecting a gallbladder issue. I didn't realize it then, but that appointment would divide my life into *before* and *after*.

The Ultrasound

The waiting room was nearly empty when I arrived that morning. Bright fluorescent lights poured over sterile white walls and outdated magazines. The space felt impersonal, like a blank canvas before something was about to be written on it. The receptionist handed me a clipboard, and I filled out the same forms I had filled out countless times for travel clearances and checkups, name, date, emergency contact, all the simple details that felt strangely fragile now.

A nurse called my name. I followed her down a narrow hallway that smelled faintly of disinfectant and lemon polish. The ultrasound room was cold and dark, lit only by the glow of a monitor. The technician greeted me warmly, her smile a small light in that dim space. She was pregnant, maybe in her late twenties, and radiated calmness. "We'll make this quick and easy," she said as I lay back on the table. Her kindness disarmed me.

The gel was cool on my skin. The transducer pressed against my abdomen, gliding methodically while the screen flickered in patterns I couldn't read. The steady hum of the machine filled the silence. I tried to make small talk, asked her how far along she was, told her I had kids too, anything to avoid the tension rising inside me.

But then she stopped talking. Her eyes narrowed slightly as she studied the monitor. "Everything okay?" I asked. She smiled faintly, the professional smile that hides concern.

She studied the monitor a second too long. "The doctor will review these images," she said. That was the moment the room got smaller. That's when I knew something else was there.

The Tests

The ultrasound confirmed a ruptured gallbladder; it would need to be removed, but it also revealed clusters of cysts on both kidneys. The doctor ordered an MRI for further evaluation. I told myself it was precautionary, but deep down, unease had already taken root.

The MRI was scheduled a few days later. I remember lying perfectly still as the machine swallowed me whole, its metallic clanking filling the narrow tube. I closed my eyes and tried to pray. *Lord, if this is something serious, give me the strength to handle it.* The noise was deafening, but the prayer felt louder inside me.

Days turned into weeks: test results, referrals, phone calls, the vocabulary of my new normal. My gallbladder surgery was scheduled for July 2007, and I went through it uneventfully, but the bigger question loomed. The MRI results showed that the cysts were widespread. My internist referred me to a nephrologist for confirmation.

The Diagnosis

By early September, I found myself driving down Sherman Avenue in New Haven, headed to **Dr. Sue Chang's** office. The street was noisy, a mix of traffic and city sounds. I remember thinking how ordinary everything looked for a day that would change everything.

The office itself was standard medical architecture, with linoleum floors, beige walls, and a small reception window. I checked in, filled out yet another form, and waited. My wife, Marcia, sat next to me, holding my hand, quiet. She had been strong through my gallbladder surgery, but I could feel her unease now.

A nurse called me in to take vitals, blood pressure, pulse, and weight, the routine before reality. Then she led us down a short corridor into Dr. Chang's office. Unlike the exam rooms, her office looked corporate, with a wood desk, framed certificates, and tidy shelves. It could have been any executive's office except for the anatomical charts on the wall.

Dr. Chang entered with a gentle nod and sat across from us. Her tone was factual, deliberate. "Daniel," she began, "your MRI confirms extensive cystic growth on both kidneys. This condition is called *Polycystic Kidney Disease,* or PKD. It's a genetic disorder. There's currently no cure."

The words hung in the air, sterile and absolute. I remember asking, trying to stay analytical, *"How long before kidney failure?"* She paused. "It's hard to predict, but probably three to five years, closer to five."

Marcia broke. Tears streamed down her face as the gravity of it sank in. I sat motionless, gripping her hand, my mind scanning for solutions the way it did when troubleshooting a system at work. *What's the root cause? What's the fix? There has to be a fix.* But this wasn't a system problem. This was me.

"You have PKD, and there's no cure."

Those words have never left me.

The Ride Home

We left Dr. Chang's office in silence. Outside, the sounds of Sherman Avenue were loud: car horns, voices, the hum of life continuing as if nothing had happened. I remember guiding Marcia toward the car, feeling her shoulders shake as she cried. Inside the car, neither of us spoke for several minutes. I gripped the steering wheel, staring straight ahead, mind blank.

Finally, I said, "We'll get through this. We'll fight it together." It was all I could offer, hope borrowed from faith, wrapped in shock.

The drive home felt longer than it was. The world looked the same, but everything was different. Every song on the radio sounded hollow, every mile an echo of uncertainty. When we pulled into the driveway, the kids were playing in the yard, their laughter piercing the haze. I forced a smile, waved, walked inside, and excused myself to the bathroom to breathe. I looked in the mirror and saw the same face, but it wasn't the same man.

That night, after we tucked the children into bed, Marcia and I sat at the kitchen table in silence. The hum of the refrigerator filled the room. "What does this mean?" she asked. I didn't know how to answer. We prayed instead, simple words, a plea for strength. *God, show us the way.*

Family & Faith

In the days that followed, we told Marcia's family. They were supportive, but I could see the worry in their eyes. I called my sister, Rose, and told her over the phone. Her reaction was strangely dismissive, maybe denial, maybe self-protection. We decided not to tell the children yet; they were too young to understand. I told a few close colleagues at Oracle, those I trusted, but otherwise kept it private. I didn't want sympathy; I wanted focus.

I immersed myself in research, learning the language of my disease: eGFR, creatinine, cyst burden, and hypertension. I realized that PKD was progressive but unpredictable. I learned to monitor sodium and potassium, to track protein intake, and to understand labs like I once understood project dashboards. Data became a kind of prayer, numbers I could measure when faith felt abstract.

But at night, when the house grew quiet, I prayed in the old-fashioned way. I asked God for time, just time to see my children grow, to keep working, to be useful. I promised to stay grateful, even if the road ahead was long.

The Inner Battle

My Navy background kicked in. When faced with adversity, you don't flinch; you plan. I treated PKD like a mission. Learn the threat. Build the defense. Stay operational. Yet this wasn't a battle fought with tactics and tools; it was fought in silence, in lab results, fatigue, and fear.

Physically, I still looked strong. My labs at that time were manageable, my eGFR in the eighties, my energy high, but the psychological shift was seismic. I began to view time differently. Every moment with my family became heavier, more sacred. Every business trip felt longer, every hug shorter.

I also wrestled with guilt, wondering if my children could inherit the same gene, if my choices had somehow accelerated what was inevitable. The mind becomes its own battlefield in those moments. But my faith, fragile but steady, kept me centered. I reminded myself that God doesn't promise a life without trials; He promises His presence through them.

Flying had shaped me long before the diagnosis. Since 1994, I have flown airplanes and helicopters, hours spent in the sky teaching me precision, patience, and respect for checklists. The Navy taught me that courage is not the absence of fear; it is the choice to keep moving when fear demands you stop. Later, serving with the Department of Defense Police in Groton, Connecticut, I learned the same quiet discipline, the same calm in uncertain moments. I also served as a volunteer firefighter in Cheshire, Connecticut, for a couple of years, where teamwork and service were not concepts; they were a way of life. I am Irish, and I can be stubborn, sometimes to my benefit and sometimes to my harm, and that stubbornness would become fuel for the long road ahead. Not having my dad around left a hole. It would have been a comfort to hear his voice, to feel his strength, to borrow a little of his steadiness while I learned to stand in my own.

Perspective Changes

My first instinct was to bury myself in work. If I kept moving, maybe the diagnosis would feel less real. I poured myself into projects, travel, and long days, and in doing so, I ignored the one thing that mattered most, my wife and my family. It was a coping strategy, and it was not a good one. I see that clearly now. Love cannot be put on hold until after the crisis. Love is the way through the crisis.

Within weeks, my daily routine changed. Medications appeared beside my toothbrush. I watched my diet, drank more water, reduced caffeine, and learned what "renal diet" truly meant. I began to decline invitations that involved long flights or late nights. I paid closer attention to my body, to the small signals I used to ignore.

But I didn't stop living. I kept teaching, working, and mentoring others. I found comfort in purpose, in the idea that my work still mattered. I wasn't going to let PKD define me; I was going to define how I lived with it.

My conversations with God deepened. I stopped treating prayer as negotiation and started treating it as dialogue. Some nights, I sat in silence, acknowledging my fear and letting grace fill the space where answers didn't exist.

Turning Point

Looking back now, that period wasn't a collapse. It was a recalibration, a shift from thinking I controlled life to realizing I was entrusted with it. PKD became my teacher. It stripped away illusions of permanence and forced me to confront what truly mattered: faith, family, service, and purpose.

The years after diagnosis brought their own trials. In 2014, I suffered a broken vertebra, another reminder that bodies have limits even when the mind insists on pushing forward. The warrior mindset and years of training carried me through the pain and through the long recovery. I chose to keep building my life rather than shrinking it. I pursued a master's degree and then a doctorate, writing papers late at night and studying between appointments. Progress was rarely dramatic. It was quiet and steady, a daily decision to keep faith, to keep learning, and to keep showing up for the people who needed me.

Through all of it, one truth crystallized in my heart: don't wait for tomorrow what you can do today. Tomorrow is only a promise, never a guarantee. That mindset changed everything for me. I realized I would rather be a *has-been* than a *could-have-been*. The sky, the sea, and even the setbacks had taught me the same lesson: life doesn't wait, and neither should we.

If I could speak to the man I was on that September day in 2007, sitting across from Dr. Chang as she said *there's no cure,* I would tell him this: "Be strong. Don't give in. Don't give up. With faith, knowledge, and courage, you'll outlast the fear. You'll work, teach, and love through it. You'll see your children grow. You'll live again, stronger, wiser, grateful."

Reflection - The Birth of Resilience

The world changed that day, but not only for the worse. What began as a diagnosis became a calling, a journey of endurance and gratitude. I learned that resilience isn't defiance; it's surrender to a greater strength. And though I didn't know it then, the same faith that steadied my hands in the Navy would one day steady me in a hospital bed waiting for a transplant.

That day in 2007 marked the end of who I thought I was, and the beginning of who I was meant to become.

Chapter 2

Understanding PKD and CKD

The day after the diagnosis, the world didn't look different, but I did. If I couldn't change the headline, I could study the footnotes. That's how the mission began: learn the system, chart the numbers, buy time. I was thirty-four, a husband and father of three, and the forecast I'd been given, three to five years, became the baseline for every decision that followed. So I turned back to what I knew best: discipline, structure, and study.

The first week after my diagnosis in 2007 was a blur of disbelief. Once the shock began to fade, I did what I have always done in the face of the unknown: I studied it. For most people, learning about a disease is optional; for me, it became survival. I wasn't just reading to understand; I was reading to live longer.

From Shock to Study

In the days after the diagnosis, the fog didn't lift all at once; it drifted upward slowly, just enough for me to see that standing still wasn't an option. I've never been someone who waits for clarity; I chase it. So I opened my laptop and began learning everything I could. Most people study an illness to feel informed. I studied mine to feel anchored. Each article and medical paper became a small foothold in a world that suddenly felt unstable.

At night, after the kids were asleep and the house was quiet, I would sit at the kitchen table with my laptop and a notebook. I started typing "Polycystic Kidney Disease" into search engines, scanning through pages from the National Institutes of Health, Mayo Clinic, and the National Kidney Foundation. I filled notebooks with terms that felt like a foreign language: nephrons, glomeruli, cystic dilation, creatinine clearance.

Slowly, science replaced fear. Each paragraph I read gave me a small measure of control back. I realized that PKD and CKD were not interchangeable; one was the cause, the other the consequence. Polycystic Kidney Disease (PKD) was the genetic blueprint that started it all, clusters of fluid-filled cysts that slowly destroyed healthy kidney tissue. Chronic Kidney Disease (CKD) was the result of the gradual loss of kidney function over time.

What I remember most from those first nights was the strange comfort in understanding the enemy. Every diagram of a kidney, every labeled artery and tubule, made the disease feel less like a shadow and more like a system, one I could learn, monitor, and influence.

What the Kidneys Really Do

Before that time, I had thought of kidneys as filters, vaguely aware that they "cleaned the blood." I didn't realize they perform a symphony of chemical and biological miracles every minute.

Each kidney, about the size of a fist, contains roughly one million microscopic filtering units called **nephrons**. These nephrons work constantly, filtering approximately 150–180 liters of blood every day and producing about one to two liters of urine. Through that process, the kidneys remove metabolic waste such as urea and creatinine, the by-products of protein metabolism, and maintain delicate balances of electrolytes like sodium, potassium, calcium, and phosphate.

But the kidneys are far more than filters. They also regulate blood pressure by releasing **renin**, stimulate red blood cell production through **erythropoietin**, and activate vitamin D for bone health. When the kidneys fail, every one of these functions begins to unravel, silently and systematically.

Learning that the kidneys control so many interlocking systems was both awe-inspiring and terrifying. I began to see my lab reports differently. Numbers that once seemed abstract, creatinine, eGFR, and BUN, now told a story. Creatinine reflected how much waste my kidneys could still clear; eGFR, my estimated filtration rate, told me roughly how much function remained.

The first time I saw my eGFR number drop below 80, I felt the gravity of it. It wasn't panic, it was purpose. Every point of decline was a reminder that I had to act smarter, eat cleaner, and live with intention.

The Science of PKD: A Genetic Blueprint

Polycystic Kidney Disease, I learned, wasn't something I had "caught." It was written into my DNA, a mutation typically on the **PKD1** or **PKD2** gene. These genes normally produce proteins that help the kidney's tubular cells maintain structure and communication. When they fail, small cysts form and multiply, gradually overtaking healthy tissue.

During that period of learning and testing, my nephrologist ordered a DNA kidney gene panel and a Renasight test to see if this came from a parent or a spontaneous mutation. The results were inconclusive, no clear family link; the working theory was a rare mutation. "Lucky me," I joked, because humor sometimes keeps the floor from giving way.

Knowing that, I started keeping a "flight log" of my own, lab values, scan dates, blood pressure readings, the way a pilot tracks altitude and fuel. The spreadsheet was cold comfort, but it gave me something to steer by.

Healthy kidneys are roughly the size of a clenched fist. In PKD, as cysts expand, each kidney can grow to the size of an **American football** (weighing up to 20–30 pounds each). When I read that, I remember putting my hand against my abdomen and whispering, "You've got to be kidding." I later confirmed through imaging that both my kidneys had indeed grown close to that scale by the time I reached the transplant stage.

I learned that cyst growth is not linear; it accelerates as the kidneys enlarge. The cysts fill with fluid, compress normal tissue, and reduce the organ's ability to filter blood. The swelling can cause abdominal fullness, back pain, and fatigue. Some patients describe it as carrying two watermelons inside their bodies. I was fortunate; I experienced discomfort but not the full physical distortion that many endure.

Emotionally, though, I carried the weight. Knowing my kidneys were expanding inside me was unsettling. Yet knowledge was still power. I began tracking my imaging results and lab values in spreadsheets. It became my flight log for survival, data, not despair.

Fear to Function: Learning the Language of Labs

I made it my mission to understand every number that appeared in my results.

- **Creatinine** measured how efficiently my kidneys removed waste; higher meant worse filtration.
- **Blood Urea Nitrogen (BUN)** indicates the amount of nitrogen in the blood from protein breakdown.
- **eGFR,** the estimated glomerular filtration rate, was the big one, a calculation that told me roughly what percentage of kidney function I had left.

I created spreadsheets that tracked each test over time. I added columns for date, creatinine, eGFR, BUN, and blood pressure. Trends became stories, some encouraging, others not. Over time, I learned that stability mattered more than a single result.

At my next nephrology appointment, I asked Dr. Chang questions that made her pause. "How exactly does the renin-angiotensin system regulate pressure when cysts distort the kidney's architecture?" She smiled and said, "You've been studying." I nodded because knowing made me less afraid.

It also gave me the conviction to challenge my own habits, particularly my diet.

Food, Fuel, and the Fragile Balance

Everything I learned about kidneys led me to the same truth: **what you eat becomes what your kidneys must handle**. The body metabolizes protein into urea and creatinine, both of which must be excreted. Sodium controls blood volume and pressure. Potassium regulates heartbeat, but, in excess, can stop it. Phosphorus builds bones but also clogs arteries if the kidneys can't filter it.

The average diet, I discovered, is a biochemical assault on fragile kidneys. Processed foods are loaded with sodium and phosphorus additives. Energy drinks and certain supplements flood the body with compounds that the kidneys must strain to remove. I began tracking everything: grams of protein, milligrams of sodium, potassium content, and even fluid ounces of water each day.

I stopped thinking of food as comfort and began seeing it as chemistry. My goal was simple: **extend beyond the three-to-five-year prognosis** Dr. Chang had given me. I wanted my kidneys to last not just a few years, but as long as humanly possible.

So I built my own "renal flight plan."

- **Protein:** moderate, about 0.6–0.8 g/kg per day, mostly from fish and plant sources.
- **Sodium:** < 2,000 mg per day to reduce pressure and swelling.

- **Potassium:** monitored carefully, especially as function declined.

- **Phosphorus:** avoided cola, processed cheese, and preserved meats.

- **Fluid:** balanced intake; neither over-hydration nor dehydration.

This wasn't about restriction; it was about precision. Every glass of water, every plate of food, became an act of stewardship.

When Knowledge Becomes Survival

The genetics of PKD made me confront more than the size of my kidneys; they challenged the future of my family. PKD is inherited in an autosomal-dominant pattern, meaning each child of a parent with the gene has a 50% chance of inheriting it. I thought of my three young children, ages four, six, and two at the time, and the weight of that probability pressed on me. Learning the biology of nephron loss, cyst proliferation, and eventual glomerular damage transformed my parental anxiety into a disciplined plan.

I charted the disease's progression step by step, the cysts forming, the kidneys enlarging, the function slowly declining, and eventually the slide into chronic kidney disease and, if left unchecked, renal failure. One clinical description stayed with me: "PKD is a genetic disorder that causes many fluid-filled cysts to grow in your kidneys. PKD is a form of CKD that reduces kidney function and may lead to kidney failure." That single sentence became a mission statement for how I approached the years ahead.

I kept that sentence in my notebook alongside lab values and action steps. I understood that CKD isn't simply an end-state; it's the process by which your body loses the ability to maintain homeostasis minute-by-minute. The first time I saw my eGFR (estimated glomerular filtration rate) drop below 80 mL/min/1.73 m², I realized this was no longer theoretical. It was real.

When the Workload Increases

I learned early that the kidneys are workhorses. They filter nearly 150 liters of blood per day, remove toxins like urea and creatinine, balance electrolytes like sodium and potassium, regulate blood pressure through renin, and stimulate red blood cell production via erythropoietin. When disease begins to erode nephron count, the remaining nephrons compensate by hyperfiltration, working harder and longer. That compensation phase can last years, masking the damage until it becomes obvious.

I recalled a late evening trip to Toronto for work, feeling subtly off. I'd dismissed the fatigue as travel-related until I looked down at the digital blood pressure cuff in my hotel room: 148/92 mmHg. That number surprised me. I realized I had been ignoring a key warning sign: hypertension is almost universal in ADPKD and can accelerate decline. I booked a nephrology consult the following week.

The physician explained: hypertension, cyst growth, and nephron loss create a "perfect storm." One of the first therapeutic goals is tight blood pressure control, to decrease glomerular damage and slow cyst expansion. I committed then to staying under 130/80 and tracking each reading. No longer an executive worried about spreadsheets alone, I became a patient committed to numbers that might determine my lifespan.

The Diet of Survival

The research on CKD taught me that diet is not optional. It is non-negotiable. Patients with CKD may need to control key nutrients: sodium, potassium, phosphorus, calcium, and protein. I made the decision: if I could control the load, maybe I could slow the decline.

Sodium. I discovered that excess sodium causes fluid retention, high blood pressure, and additional strain on my kidneys. I wrote: *Keep sodium ≤ 2,000 mg/day.* I began reading labels, comparing brands, and adopting herbs instead of salt. A 2022 guideline review suggested < 2 g/day sodium (~5 g salt) for adults with CKD. I adopted that as a target.

Protein. The kidneys must clear waste produced from protein breakdown, especially urea and creatinine. In my spreadsheets, I tracked protein grams per kilogram bodyweight: for kidney preservation, many sources recommend ~0.8 g/kg/day for CKD stages 1-3. I weighed 85 kg; I aimed for ~68 g protein/day. That felt like a challenge for a man used to going to the gym three times a week, but I accepted it.

Potassium. The balance of potassium is critical; too much can cause arrhythmias, and too little impacts muscle and heart function. I learned that as kidney function declines, serum potassium rises unless intake is restricted or clearance improved. I created a list of "high potassium" foods to limit: bananas, potatoes, beans, and dairy, while ensuring my diet remained satisfying.

Phosphorus & Calcium. Later, I would add these to my tracking when my labs showed an upward trend. However, early on, I avoided colas, processed meats, and cheese-heavy meals, knowing phosphorus additives were a silent stress on failing kidneys.

Fluid Intake. I learned that neither overhydration nor dehydration is wise. The kidneys must manage volume; too much and the heart swells, too little and the kidneys suffer. In my travel days, I always had a large water bottle; now I treated water like fuel. I drank water, but monitored weight, swelling, and blood pressure daily.

The Symphony Within

When I first began studying the kidneys, I was struck not just by their biology but by their elegance. Millions of nephrons work in silence, regulating chemistry and pressure with tireless precision. I had once thought of kidneys as simple filters; now I saw them as a living symphony, intricate, purposeful, and awe-inspiring. Learning their design didn't just educate me; it humbled me. Even in illness, the body carried a kind of quiet brilliance.

It humbled me. I used to think of the kidneys simply as waste filters, plumbing for the body. What I learned was that they are more like silent air-traffic controllers, coordinating the chemistry of life second-by-second: managing pH, regulating blood pressure through **renin**, signaling the bone marrow to produce red blood cells through **erythropoietin**, and activating vitamin D for calcium absorption. They are less mechanical than symphonic.

Metabolism and the Hidden Load

Understanding metabolism through the lens of CKD was eye-opening. Every time we eat, drink, or move, we create metabolic by-products: nitrogen from protein, acid from digestion, and electrolytes from every cellular process. Healthy kidneys clear them effortlessly. Diseased kidneys, however, begin to struggle.

I began to visualize each meal as a chemical equation:

- **Protein** → urea + ammonia

- **Potassium** ↑ → cardiac strain

- **Sodium** ↑ → blood-pressure load

- **Phosphorus** ↑ → bone demineralization

When my labs first showed a mild rise in creatinine, my instinct was not panic; it was curiosity. I spent nights reading research papers, some from the *National Center for Biotechnology Information*, learning how reduced glomerular filtration allows toxins to linger in the bloodstream. The more I understood, the more empowered I felt. Knowledge became medicine.

I also learned why doctors emphasize protein moderation: breaking down dietary protein produces nitrogenous waste, which the kidneys must excrete as urea. For someone with CKD, this extra workload can accelerate decline. I began viewing my plate not as a restriction but as optimization, fuel management for longevity.

Symptoms Beyond Numbers

Numbers tell one story; the body tells another. Fatigue became my first subtle messenger. Some mornings, it felt as though I would run a marathon overnight. Later, I learned that reduced erythropoietin production can lead to anemia, a shortage of red blood cells that saps oxygen and energy.

Occasionally, I would notice a faint metallic or ammonia-like taste in my mouth. At first, I thought it was dental or dietary. In truth, it was a trace of **uremic buildup**, toxins the kidneys could no longer clear completely. The National Kidney Foundation describes this as a common early warning sign of CKD progression.

I also paid attention to subtle swelling in my ankles during long flights. The kidneys regulate fluid balance, and even slight inefficiencies can lead to fluid accumulation. Small details became data points in my self-study.

Despite these physiological reminders, I remained active. I still lectured, led projects, and exercised within reason. I refused to surrender vitality to diagnosis. The key was adjusting the rhythm, not quitting the song.

When the Mind Joins the Fight

The greatest challenge was not physical; it was mental. I realized that CKD is a slow-burning illness, and the mind can grow restless waiting for the body to "fail." That tension, the waiting, the uncertainty, became its own test of faith.

During those years, I adopted a rule: *action over anxiety.* If fear visited, I countered it with knowledge. If fatigue arrived, I met it with gratitude. My faith played a huge role in this reframing. I found peace in Scriptures like Isaiah 41:10, "Do not fear, for I am with you." I wrote those words on a Post-it and stuck it to my bathroom mirror. Each morning, it reminded me that my health was not a punishment but a pilgrimage.

My conversations with doctors evolved from reactive to collaborative. Instead of asking "What can't I do?" I asked, "What can I optimize?" They appreciated the engagement. I think part of healing is reclaiming agency; even small choices, a meal, a walk, a prayer, feel like victories.

What I Learned About Balance

The human body operates on equilibrium, and nowhere is that more evident than in kidney physiology, where sodium and potassium dance opposites: one pulling water in, the other pushing it out. Calcium and phosphorus shape our bones, but can harden our arteries when imbalanced. Even water, the simplest molecule, becomes both healer and harm depending on the dose.

So, I learned to **respect moderation as discipline**, not deprivation. Each time I said no to excess salt or skipped an extra coffee, I imagined I was buying another day of function, another sunrise to see my kids grow.

In this quiet practice of balance, I found something deeper: grace. My kidneys, though scarred and enlarged, still worked. Every lab that came back "stable" felt like an answered prayer. The doctors gave me 3 to 5 years. Through vigilance, diet, and faith, I surpassed that many times over.

Action Over Anxiety

Chronic illness teaches you that waiting is never passive. It can gnaw at you, whisper worst-case scenarios, and leave you frozen in the space between what is and what might be. To stay steady, I built a simple rule: do something. If fear tried to pull me into the future, I brought myself back to the present with action, even small action. A cleaned-up diet. A logged blood pressure. A question prepared for my next appointment.

Over time, this approach reshaped how I spoke with my doctors. Instead of focusing on what was slipping out of my hands, I focused on what still belonged to me: my habits, my preparation, my attitude. A stable lab, a day without swelling, a successful walk around the block, these became wins.

I eventually learned that healing is not only about medicine or metrics. Sometimes the act of moving, learning, adjusting, even in small ways, is its own form of strength. Action became my anchor.

What Balance Taught Me

The body is built on opposites that must stay in harmony: sodium and potassium, calcium and phosphorus, work and rest. Even water, life's simplest element, becomes harmful in excess. Moderation turned from nuisance to discipline, a spiritual practice disguised as a diet.

Each small act of restraint felt like buying another day, another sunrise, another chance to see my children grow.

Reflection – From Knowledge to Grace

Understanding PKD and CKD was never just about biology; it was about perspective. The more I learned about the body, the more I saw evidence of both science and spirit working in tandem. Each nephron became a reminder that life's systems are fragile but purposeful. Every stable lab result felt like a minor miracle earned through vigilance and mercy.

Over the years, I came to realize that this process, the research, the note-taking, the endless reading, was an education unto itself. It was not formal, but it was essential. It was the curriculum of survival, one I had not chosen but had to master. I viewed it as my second doctorate, not in data or leadership, but in life itself.

That education became a lifeline. It taught me to measure progress not only in numbers but in faith, in patience, in gratitude. It reminded me that every decision, what to eat, how to rest, when to pray, was an act of stewardship over the life I had been given.

In the end, I learned that knowledge, when guided by purpose, becomes grace. Moreover, that grace, the union of science, discipline, and faith, became the foundation of my continuity, my best chance, and my quiet victory over the odds.

Chapter 3

Living Under the Shadow

The day eventually came when research could no longer insulate me from reality. I had learned the chemistry, the genes, the lab values, but knowledge, I discovered, is lighter than the weight of living with what you know. Understanding PKD had given me clarity; living with it demanded courage.

As one line I once heard reminded me: "The measure of a person's strength isn't in what they lift, but in what they carry quietly."

And so began the long season of carrying through work, through faith, through every morning that asked for steadiness more than strength.

The War Within (2006 – 2008)

When I look back at the years just before and after my diagnosis, I see a younger man standing unknowingly at the edge of a long, invisible war.

The pain began around 2005, dull, persistent, and strangely personal. I blamed it on stress, on travel, on long days behind a screen and longer nights of ambition. Like most people with busy lives and hidden worries, I explained away the discomfort: bad food, tension, or age. But deep down, I sensed something wasn't right.

By 2006, the pain sharpened into an ache that reached beneath the ribs and never quite released its grip. Tests led to my gallbladder surgery, a supposed fix, but even afterward, a residue of pain remained. It was as though my body was whispering a warning I didn't yet understand.

In 2007, I walked into Dr. Chang's office on Sherman Avenue in New Haven. The waiting room was bright and sterile, half-empty, filled with the quiet hum of an air vent and the faint traffic noise from the street. The neighborhood was loud and working-class, the kind of place where life moved fast, indifferent to anyone's private fear. Inside, however, time slowed.

After vitals and blood pressure, I was led into a smaller exam room. Dr. Chang entered, professional, steady, her tone matter-of-fact. She explained the imaging results and then said words that rearranged my life:

"You have Polycystic Kidney Disease. There's no treatment. No cure."

It didn't sound like a diagnosis; it sounded like a sentence. I remember nodding as if acknowledging a military order. My wife,

Marcia, beside me, began to cry softly. I reached for her hand and said what I believed at that moment: "We'll get through this."

But inside, my mind had already shifted into combat mode. This is war, I thought. Collect intelligence. Define objectives. Execute the mission. Survival is the primary goal.

Fear didn't paralyze me; it structured me. The Navy had trained me to function under stress, to rely on systems and plans. So I built one: research, monitor, adapt. I spent evenings reading medical journals, bookmarking websites, filling notebooks with terminology I could barely pronounce, such as nephrons, glomeruli, cystic dilation, and creatinine clearance.

Each fact was a weapon against helplessness.

Still, the shadow was heavy. At night, after the children went to bed, I sometimes drowned the silence in whiskey at the Irish American Home, a refuge of laughter, music, and belonging. There I could pretend for a few hours that nothing was wrong. I told myself I was managing stress, but truthfully, I was drinking to mute the echo of mortality.

Those early years were a paradox: the body breaking down, the will hardening. I revised my diet, limited sodium and potassium, worked out when I could, but carried the fatigue of sleepless nights and old grief. The loss of my parents years earlier, and the unseen weight of service-related trauma, had never been fully exorcised. I later realized that what I called "restlessness" was likely undiagnosed PTSD.

Marcia's fear ran deeper than mine. Her emotions surfaced quickly, then settled into quiet endurance. Once the initial shock passed, life resumed, birthday parties, school pickups, work deadlines, as though normalcy could will the disease away. The kids were still small, unaware of the battle unfolding beneath the surface.

Through it all, I stayed composed. That composure wasn't denial; it was discipline. Every lab report, every new test, was another mission update. My eGFR hovered within normal limits, but I knew what was coming. Doctors said three to five years before renal failure. I intended to triple that.

And in the stillness of early mornings, coffee brewing, the house quiet, I repeated a silent creed: Discipline beats despair.

Under Orders and Under Fire (2008)

In 2008, not even a year after hearing the word incurable, I found myself flying east again, not for leisure, but for duty. Oracle had been awarded a strategic contract with the U.S. Department of Defense and the Business Transformation Agency (BTA) to modernize enterprise and financial governance systems across the

Middle East. The project demanded security clearances, precision, and a tolerance for uncertainty, qualities my Navy background had already forged.

At the time, I was still serving in the U.S. Navy Reserves. That dual identity, civilian leader by day, naval sailor by oath, often placed me in spaces where responsibility outweighed comfort. It wasn't combat duty, just advisory and consultancy. Still, it carried the same expectations: discipline, precision, and the quiet understanding that your decisions mattered. That background became the lens through which I approached every mission, including this one.

I first went to Amman, Jordan, working with the Central Bank to align ERP and compliance protocols with regional efforts. From there, I was assigned to Forward Operating Base Falcon and Forward Operating Base Warhorse, on the outskirts of Baghdad, where Oracle-driven systems supported logistics, finance, and accountability overlays under combat conditions. At the time, I held TS/SCI clearance, while still serving in the U.S. Navy Reserves, a dual-hatted status that allowed me to operate both as a civilian consultant and as an officer, translating enterprise logic into mission survival.

I remember the first flight into Baghdad International Airport vividly. At altitude, the cabin fell silent except for the engines' whine. Then came the approach, a steep, corkscrewing descent designed to minimize exposure to RPGs, small-arms fire, and MANPADS from the ground. The plane banked sharply, the horizon spinning in tight circles. You could feel the shift from commercial calm to combat precision. The descent ended with a hard landing, followed by the quick taxi into the secure perimeter. Welcome to Baghdad.

The FOB was austere, with Hesco walls, dust that clung to everything, and the constant percussion of distance and danger. I remember the Route Irish we took from the Green Zone to Baghdad's airport, a partly unpaved convoy corridor infamous for IEDs and ambushes. We called it the Irish Express, half-joke, half-warning. The road wound past burned-out vehicles, checkpoints, and the smell of metal and heat. Every trip felt like rolling the dice with fate.

On one of those runs, our convoy came to an abrupt halt. Word came down that elements had been spotted on the road ahead. For nearly forty-five minutes, maybe an hour, we waited in the stifling heat, engines idling, eyes scanning the horizon. Finally, the EOD team arrived in an MRAP, methodically approaching the suspected site. Then came the controlled detonation, a deep, concussive boom that rattled through your chest. The blast marked both relief and reminder: every mile in and out of Baghdad was borrowed time.

Inside the perimeter, the work continued relentlessly. PowerPoint by day, indirect fire by night. I watched young soldiers and contractors shoulder impossible tasks with stoic humor. One young Marine, barely twenty, told me, "Sir, this is where governance meets grit." He was right. We weren't just implementing software; we were helping an exhausted system stand again.

IED detonations punctuated the horizon often enough to become background noise. I met men and women who had already served multiple tours. One old contractor, a seasoned operator from Nebraska, training Iraqi Police, looked at me and said, "You'll be back. We all do." His words lingered longer than the echo of any explosion.

After a time of rotation between Amman and Baghdad, the mission concluded. I boarded a seventeen-hour flight from the desert to Detroit, then another to Hartford. From there, I drove straight to Cape Cod, where my family was vacationing. The contrast was surreal, waves instead of sirens, my children running on sand instead of soldiers walking through sandstorms.

When I hugged Marcia on that beach, I realized the deployment had closed something in me, not just exhaustion, but an emotional loop between duty and mortality. I had seen enough war to know that life is both fragile and deliberate.

That journey, across continents and combat zones, became more than a return home. It was a return to purpose.

Hiding in Plain Sight (2009 – 2015)

By 2009, I had become adept at secrecy. My résumé grew, my leadership roles expanded, but so did the quiet rituals of illness, lab appointments, imaging scans, and medication refills. Few colleagues knew. I wore my professionalism like armor, concealing weakness not out of pride, but out of instinct.

At Oracle and later at Yale, the workload was relentless. I met deadlines, led teams, lectured, and traveled, all while my kidneys silently expanded inside me. When fatigue struck mid-afternoon, I drank black coffee, smiled through it, and pressed on. The Navy had a phrase for this: embrace the suck. I did.

I remember rolling down my shirt sleeves to hide blood-draw tape before walking into meetings. I'd sit across from executives, discuss enterprise systems, and no one could see that my abdomen throbbed with a low, internal pressure. The illusion of normalcy was its own strange comfort.

But concealment has a cost. The body whispers before it screams. Headaches became routine. My blood pressure crept upward, sometimes 140/90, 150/95, numbers I dismissed until one night in a Toronto hotel, alone after a long workday, I checked my pressure on a travel monitor: 148/92. That glow of red digits against the dark hotel room felt like a warning flare.

Hypertension, I later learned, is nearly universal in ADPKD and accelerates decline. The realization was sobering. I booked an appointment with Dr. Chang that same week. She confirmed what I feared: the kidneys were compensating, hyper-filtering to make up for lost nephrons. "Control your pressure," she said. "That's your front line."

From then on, I tracked it obsessively. 130/80 became a mission parameter. I charted each reading in Excel, alongside creatinine, BUN, and eGFR. The spreadsheet looked like flight data, each line a new sortie in a long campaign.

Through these years, my faith re-entered quietly. Between 2011 and 2013, I began attending Mass again, sometimes daily. The church became a kind of command center for the soul, no noise, no metrics, only presence. In confession, I spoke less about sins and more about surrender. I remember telling a priest, "I'm not afraid to die, Father. I'm afraid to stop living before I die." He nodded gently and said, "Then don't."

Faith gave me a new framework. I no longer prayed for miracles; I prayed for stamina.

Marcia adapted too. Where she once panicked, she now steadied. We rarely spoke of the disease, not out of avoidance, but because we understood each other without needing many words. PKD hovered in the background, acknowledged but not allowed to dominate our lives. Our children were growing, eleven, nine, and seven by 2012, and they needed stability more than medical explanations.

In 2014, life delivered an unexpected blow. While trimming a large tree behind the house, I slipped from a ladder nearly thirty feet high. The fall was instantaneous. The landing was violent. I remember the sound of impact, the air rushing out of my lungs, and the strange stillness afterward as I lay staring up at the sky. I wiggled my toes to make sure I hadn't lost them. When the paramedics arrived, I insisted on walking to the stretcher—a stubborn act of defiance that made no medical sense but felt necessary in the moment.

At the ER, scans revealed a burst fracture at L3. Dr. Waitze examined me and said, "No fusion needed. You're going to walk again." He helped me stand, and though every nerve screamed, I took three unsteady steps. Those steps felt like resurrection. I spent a week in rehab and returned to work soon after, wrapped in a bulky back brace that made me look like a turtle, slow but unstoppable.

That accident humbled me. It reminded me that survival isn't just a mindset; it's grace.

By the time 2015 arrived, I was managing six daily medications, juggling blood draws, imaging, and teaching. Fatigue was constant, but I refused to let it rewrite my identity. Even colleagues who knew about my diagnosis were often surprised at how active I remained. I maintained composure, led teams, and even trained others. Still, privately, I slept longer, prayed harder, and thanked God for every stable lab result.

Two years after my 2014 incident, in 2016, another loss cut even deeper. My brother Jim's cancer returned. He fought with quiet courage until the end, and his passing in Philadelphia felt like a wound that reached all the way down to the bone. Standing beside his hospital bed, I saw not only my brother but a mirror, another man wrestling with faith, time, and the body's fragility. Losing him rekindled my own fear of the clock, the slow tick of a disease that gave no promises.

Living under the shadow no longer meant fear of the dark. It meant learning how to see in low light, to sense the presence of hope even when certainty was gone.

And so I carried on, half-warrior, half-pilgrim, aware that the battle was far from over, yet convinced that the mission was still mine to complete.

The Quiet Fire (2015 – 2020)

By 2015, something within me shifted quietly, almost imperceptibly at first. After nearly a decade of managing PKD like an enemy, I began to see it as a reluctant teacher. The battle continued, yes, but the posture changed. I was no longer fighting *against* life; I was learning how to live *within* it.

Professionally, my trajectory kept climbing. I moved from Yale to Quinnipiac University as Chief Technology Officer, then later to corporate leadership roles that demanded both precision and endurance. Outwardly, I was thriving, building teams, leading digital transformation projects, and advising senior executives. Inwardly, I was recalibrating what success meant.

Teaching became the turning point. Standing before students, translating analytics and algorithms into human terms, I discovered something sacred in the exchange. The classroom wasn't only about instruction; it was about connection, about purpose. I realized that every hour spent mentoring young minds was an hour I wasn't thinking about disease.

At first, I thought I was teaching *them*. Over time, I understood they were teaching *me* patience, empathy, and the quiet fire that keeps hope alive.

Evenings that once revolved around lab results and medication schedules began to share space with grading papers and advising projects. Those students, future data scientists, analysts, and cybersecurity specialists, didn't know that their professor went home each night with kidneys the size of footballs. They only saw enthusiasm, rigor, and humor. And maybe that was the point: life, when shared, is lighter to carry.

An Unexpected Sister (2017)

By early 2017, life felt strangely balanced. My faith was steady, my career intense, my teaching deeply fulfilling. The kids were growing, and Marcia and I had found a rhythm that carried us through the long, quiet years of PKD's slow advance.

And then, without warning, life delivered a gift I had waited decades to receive.

Growing up, I always knew I had an older half-sister on my father's side. Her name was Kathleen. A name spoken gently, rarely, almost reverently. She was a part of my father's past that never fully crossed into the present. I spent years searching, old phone books, rumors, and family threads that ended abruptly. Always wanting to find her. Never succeeding.

Then one afternoon, I opened the Ancestry DNA app and felt my heart skip.

A new match.

A close match.

Immediate family.

I stared at the screen, hardly breathing. There it was, a connection I had dreamed of but never expected to see.

Her surname was different now, so I wasn't entirely sure. But something in me said, *try*. So I drafted an email, simple, humble, hopeful, and pressed send, fully expecting it to vanish into the quiet void where so many earlier attempts had gone.

That weekend, I drove to my sister-in-law's lake house, where Marcia and her sisters were gathered. Standing by the water, almost sheepish, I said, "I think I finally found Kathleen."

Marcia gave the kindest smile, the kind people offer when they want to protect your heart. "That would be great," she said, "but let's not get our hopes up."

Fair. I had hoped before.

But later that night, after we returned home, I checked my email on my phone.

There it was, **her reply**.

That email became a conversation. Then a relationship. And when she sent a photo, I remember feeling something inside me shift. The resemblance was uncanny: the face shape, the eyes, the unmistakable O'Connell imprint.

It was like seeing a missing chapter of myself suddenly appear.

We began speaking regularly. She was gracious, warm, welcoming, and curious about the brother she never knew she had. And I felt a healing I didn't realize I'd been waiting for.

Finding Kathleen wasn't just a moment of connection; it was a quiet kind of restoration.

A reminder that not everything we lose stays lost...
and not all prayers are answered quickly, but some are answered perfectly.

In a year when my health would soon begin to decline more noticeably, God placed someone in my life who reminded me of who I was and where I came from, before illness tried to define me.

Building and Rebuilding

In 2013, we had moved to a new house in Cheshire, and by 2015, home improvement became therapy. I built a basement office with my own hands, finished the walls, installed lighting, and added a spare bedroom. Every nail driven was a declaration: *I am still capable.*

Later came the deck. Then the pool. Each project became a dialogue with time: how much could I build before the next setback?

PKD teaches patience. Wood teaches the same. You can't rush structure.

Those years also became about restoring what I had once endangered: my marriage, my family's peace, and my own sense of grace. The affair years earlier had left cracks in everything stable. Through counseling, prayer, and accountability, Marcia and I rebuilt trust slowly. There was forgiveness, but not amnesia. The disease made honesty unavoidable; it stripped away illusions until only truth remained.

We began spending more evenings together again, quiet dinners, family movies, and road trips to Cape Cod and other parts of New England. The kids were growing fast, their laughter returning to the house like sunlight.

Pain and Purpose

Physically, the symptoms evolved. The pain in my flanks grew dull but constant, like a low drumbeat under the day. Some mornings, putting on a belt required care, a subtle reminder that space inside me was shrinking.

But it wasn't just the body that hurt. Fatigue could flatten me without warning. One moment I'd be lecturing with energy; the next, I'd feel gravity double its weight. Still, I refused to surrender motion. I taught standing up. I spoke with momentum. I smiled even when my breath was shallow.

Occasionally, I felt cysts rupture, a stabbing internal pressure followed by nausea. The episodes passed, but they reinforced the reality: the enemy was within, patient and persistent.

And yet, I saw beauty even in biology. I studied nephron structure the way I once studied flight manuals, every diagram, every term. The kidneys' complexity humbled me. How could something so intricate betray itself? It reminded me of systems I built at work: one flaw in code, one failed node, and the entire network falters.

I began to talk about resilience in lectures, not explicitly about my illness, but through data analogies. "In every system," I'd tell students, "redundancy and recovery matter more than perfection." What they didn't know was that I was describing myself.

By 2019, I had achieved what most people call stability. My eGFR hovered in the 30s, declining but consistent. My faith deepened. My family was stronger. And my sense of purpose, to teach, to lead, to serve, burned steadier than ever.

Still, the numbers didn't lie. The countdown had begun.

The Countdown (2020 – 2023)

The world changed in 2020, and so did I.

When COVID hit, isolation became the new normal. For someone with compromised kidneys, isolation wasn't just recommended; it was mandatory. I worked from home, taught remotely, and watched society retreat behind screens. Strangely, the solitude suited me. I had spent years living in my own form of quarantine, careful, measured, waiting.

By 2023, my eGFR slipped into the 20s, the line between chronic and critical. I felt it long before the numbers confirmed it: the heaviness in my body, the metallic edge of uremia on my tongue, the swelling in my ankles after long days. When my nephrologist finally said, gently and directly, 'It's time to start thinking about transplant,' it wasn't a surprise. But it still landed with weight.

The words didn't shock me this time. They invited preparation.

I had outlived every prognosis, 13 years post-diagnosis, still dialysis-free. Gratitude and fear mingled like old companions. I knew the path ahead: tests, evaluations, waiting lists, insurance forms, and the prolonged uncertainty of donor matching.

Through it all, faith became my compass. I began each morning in prayer: "Lord, if this is the time, prepare the way. Keep me steady. Keep me thankful."

I read Scripture differently now, not as distant lessons, but as survival codes. Isaiah 41:10 returned often: *"Do not fear, for I am with you; do not be dismayed, for I am your God."* Those words felt written for the transplant floor.

Beyond The Pandemic Years

COVID reshaped medicine, telehealth visits, masked interactions, and sterilized distance. Yet it also reshaped gratitude. Every breath became an act of thanksgiving.

I watched the world wrestle with mortality on a global scale and thought, *Now they know*. Everyone was living under a shadow of uncertainty, much like kidney patients do every day. For once, the fragility of life was not hidden behind routine.

Despite the chaos, my own care continued. Dr. Chang and the Hartford Hospital transplant team guided me through testing. I was listed officially in February 2024, but the process began long before, including labs, imaging, cardiac clearance, and psychological evaluations. I treated it like flight prep: each check a box to stay airborne.

My wife's anxiety resurfaced during this time. She watched me with quiet vigilance, every cough, every moment of fatigue. We prayed together nightly. Sometimes we said nothing, just held hands and listened to the house breathe around us.

Teaching persisted, even online. My students saw only a professor with good lighting and calm explanations. They didn't know that, between lectures, I checked lab results, and that I had a standing bag half-packed in case the call came.

The Call

The call came on an ordinary day.

It was May 2024, a weekday afternoon. My phone lit up with a number from Hartford Hospital. I expected a scheduling update. Instead, the coordinator's voice was steady but electric:

"Dan, we're scheduling your transplant. You have a donor."

I froze. The air felt thick. For a moment, I couldn't speak. Gratitude and disbelief tangled together.

Days later, my friend and colleague Ryan called me privately. His voice was calm, humble. "It's me," he said. "I'm your donor."

I was stunned. This was no abstract match; this was someone I worked alongside, laughed with, and strategized with. Ryan was fifteen years younger, healthy, and determined. The genetic compatibility was nearly perfect.

The surgery date, September 4, 2024, exactly seventeen years to the day of my diagnosis, felt less like a coincidence than choreography.

In those months of waiting, I prayed daily for Ryan's safety, for my family's peace, for the surgeons' hands. My eGFR had dropped to 7 by early September, but I still wasn't on dialysis, an extraordinary gift in itself.

I told my students the week before the operation. The room fell still, some gasped, others nodded in quiet solidarity. Later that night, one emailed: "Professor, thank you for teaching us that strength isn't the absence of fear."

I read it twice, then smiled. That message became what I thought was going to be my final lecture note of the semester.

The Light Beyond the Shadow (2024 – 2025)

The morning of surgery arrived before dawn.

I remember the sterile chill of Hartford Hospital, the hum of monitors, the rhythm of footsteps echoing down the hall. Ryan was already being prepped when I arrived at 6 a.m. The nurse drew what felt like gallons of blood; the anesthesiologist explained the sequence; Marcia sat beside me, eyes red but steady.

Before they wheeled me to the OR, we held hands. "I'll see you soon," I said. "I know," she whispered.

Then the mask, the countdown, ten, nine, eight, and darkness.

Six hours later, light. The blurred sound of machines. A voice asking, "Daniel, can you hear me?" I could. The first sensation was not pain, but gratitude. My body felt foreign yet alive.

That night in the ICU, I drifted between sleep and awareness. Compression sleeves hissed softly around my legs. The monitor beeped in measured rhythm. I stared at the ceiling and whispered, "Thank You."

By morning, I learned the new kidney had taken immediately, 60 eGFR within hours. The lab sheet felt like resurrection data.

Later that day, with assistance, I walked. It wasn't graceful, but it was movement, the kind I had fought to preserve for nearly two decades.

Before evening, I visited Ryan's room. He looked pale but calm. "You okay?" I asked. He smiled weakly. "Better than you, I think." We both laughed, even as guilt washed over me. He had given me part of his life so I could continue mine. How do you ever repay that?

In the days that followed, he struggled more than I did, with pain, fatigue, and the donor's burden. I recovered quickly, walking halls by day 2, and was discharged by day 5. My gratitude was indescribable.

Rebuilding a New Normal

At home, I created a new spreadsheet for diet, medications, lab values, blood pressure, and weight. Discipline was comfort. Each cell represented the control regained.

Within three weeks, I was teaching online again; by week four, back on campus. The doctors cautioned rest; I countered with reasoned defiance. *Slow is smooth, smooth is fast,* the Navy had taught me. Recovery wasn't a race; it was precision.

Each sunrise carried new clarity. Food tasted sharper. The air smelled cleaner. The fatigue that had haunted me for years dissolved into a quiet energy. The simple act of urinating, something most take for granted, became holy.

Ryan and I kept in touch constantly. Our friendship deepened, bound now by blood and sacrifice. I told him once, "You didn't just give me a kidney; you gave my kids their father back."

By 2025, life had stabilized. My labs were strong, my work fulfilling, my faith unshakable. The scars remained, both visible and unseen, but they no longer symbolized loss. They marked victory.

Reflection – Living Through the Shadow

Eighteen years.

That's how long it's been since I first heard Dr. Chang say, "There's no cure." I've lived almost two decades under that shadow, and yet, it never truly darkened me. It shaped me.

At first, *living under the shadow* meant survival, the constant vigilance of numbers, pills, and fear. Over time, it became something different: stewardship. Understanding that every breath, every heartbeat, every student taught or child hugged, is borrowed light.

I've learned that courage isn't found in loud declarations but in quiet continuance. It's in showing up for work after a sleepless night. It's in forgiving yourself for the mistakes you made when you were scared. It's in believing that purpose can coexist with pain.

Science kept me alive. Faith kept me whole. Together they formed a covenant of logic and grace.

Today, my transplanted kidney hums quietly beneath my ribs, a living reminder that miracles often arrive through human hands. I track my labs, yes, but I also track gratitude.

If there's one truth I'd leave for anyone living under their own shadow, it's this: You can't always choose the burden, but you can decide how to carry it.

And sometimes, carrying it with faith, knowledge, and love becomes the very light that outshines the shadow.

A New Chapter of Purpose (2025)

Recovery did more than restore my body; it rearranged my priorities. Once the initial months of healing settled into a quiet rhythm, I felt a stirring inside me, a sense that this second chance required something from me. Not repayment, because how do you repay a miracle? But stewardship. Purpose.

I had begun my doctoral work years earlier, slowly, steadily, through hospital appointments, teaching semesters, and the long decline of kidney function. Many people pursue a doctorate to advance their careers. I pursued it, in part, to prove something to myself, that PKD would not define the borders of my ambition, that illness would not have the last word on my future.

Finishing it during recovery was never the plan. But grace rarely consults our calendars.

Through the fall of 2025, while still tracking labs and attending checkups, I completed the final revisions of my dissertation. I wrote in early mornings with coffee steaming beside me, and late at night when the house settled into silence. Each paragraph felt like stitching a new identity, no longer a man bracing against a countdown, but a man rebuilding with deliberate intention.

Then came November.

I joined my dissertation defense wearing the quiet confidence of someone who had already survived the most challenging test. The committee greeted me warmly, unaware of the journey that had carried me there: the surgeries, the prayers, the spreadsheets, the years of teaching while kidneys failed silently beneath my ribs.

For ninety minutes, I presented my research on AI governance, education, ethics, and leadership. This subject had become personal in ways academia could not quantify. When the questions ended and the committee stepped out, I sat alone for a moment, breathing. A year earlier, I had questioned if I would live long enough to finish this degree. Now I was sitting upright, strong, speaking clearly, with another man's kidney working quietly inside me.

When they returned, they were smiling.

"Congratulations, Dr. O'Connell. You have successfully defended."

The title didn't feel like an accolade; it felt like an affirmation. A marker that the long shadow had not defeated me. That purpose had outpaced pain that the kid from Staten Island, who once carried fear and quiet wars inside him, could still rise into something new.

I walked out into the cold November air feeling lighter than I had in years. The world seemed sharper, brighter, almost freshly drawn. And for the first time in a long time, I didn't feel like I was living under a shadow.

I felt like I was living beyond it.

Reflection – Learning to See in Low Light

Living under the shadow taught me that strength is rarely loud. For nearly two decades, I carried a quiet war inside me while life went on around me, meetings, flights, classrooms, kids' birthdays, home projects, and even days spent near a war zone. On the surface, I was the executive, the professor, the Navy officer, the husband and father who "had it together." Beneath it, lab values were trending the wrong way, headaches, blood pressure creeping up, kidneys silently expanding, and memories from service that never fully stood down. PKD didn't just test my body; it tested my definitions of courage, identity, and purpose. Over time, I realized that courage wasn't charging into danger; it was getting up on an ordinary Tuesday, putting on a shirt over fresh tape from a blood draw, and choosing to lead, teach, and love anyway.

The shadow never fully disappeared, but it changed meaning. At first, it felt like a sentence; later, it became a teacher. It taught me to live deliberately, to find grace in small rituals, Mass in a quiet chapel, building a basement office with my own hands, sharing a joke with a student, and hearing my kids' laughter drift through the house. It forced honesty in my marriage, depth in my faith, and a different kind of empathy for people fighting battles no one can see. I learned that you don't wait for the shadow to lift before you live; you learn how to live *within* it, guided by faith, discipline, and love. Also, in that dim light, I discovered something unexpected: even when certainty is gone, hope still knows the way forward.

II

The Long Decline

Chapter 4

Daily Life with CKD/PKD

By the time the dust of those early battles settled, life didn't end; it recalibrated. The war had shifted from explosions and headlines to numbers and routines. In 2008, I returned home not just from deployment, but from denial. That year marked the quiet beginning of the long stretch of living with chronic kidney disease and the relentless discipline it required.

Each morning began the same way: coffee brewing, laptop on, lab results in my mind before I even checked them. PKD had taught me to live by numbers, creatinine, BUN, eGFR, potassium, and hemoglobin. They weren't just medical data points; they were coordinates in a survival map. I learned to navigate by them as instinctively as I once did by stars or instruments in a cockpit.

For the first few years after diagnosis, lab work came every other month. A metabolic panel, a CBC with auto-differential, and sometimes a 24-hour urine test every six months. Those early results gave me enough to plan between storms. But as the years progressed, the tempo quickened. By the time I neared transplant evaluation, labs had become the rule of the day: weekly bloodwork, countless vials, a blur of ECGs, MRIs, stress tests, and consultations.
It felt at times as if my life was measured in milliliters.

Dr. Chang remained a constant through it all, steady, pragmatic, and unsentimental in the best possible way. In the early years, I saw her every six months; by year ten, our meetings became quarterly. As my numbers declined, she guided me toward the next reality: Yale for transplant evaluation, then the VA, then Hartford Hospital. Each center had its own rhythm and requirements, but the goal was the same: to secure the lifeline before the inevitable.

Between tests, I tried to live like everything was fine. I traveled, lectured, led teams, and built systems. I was determined to live an everyday life, even if "normal" had changed its definition. I wore professionalism like armor. No one needed to know how much effort it took to look effortless.

The Routine

Diet came next. For the first five years, I made a few changes, still enjoyed coffee, a typical mix of meals, and occasional indulgences. But around 2012, when the disease began asserting itself, I tightened the reins. Out went the sodium and heavy proteins; in came hydration logs, fluid targets, and calculated restraint. I limited potassium, watched phosphorus, and drank more water than I thought humanly possible. Earl Grey tea became my quiet indulgence until post-transplant, when I had to give it up entirely. The irony wasn't lost on me; the tea I'd adopted for calm was suddenly off-limits in the new life I had fought for.

Food became fuel, not comfort. There's a discipline in every sip and swallow when you know your chemistry depends on it. And yet, that discipline gave me control. I couldn't cure PKD, but I could manage it, refine it, engineer my days to outsmart the clock.

The Body's Demands

The pain was unpredictable. Sometimes dull and bearable, other times sharp enough to stop me mid-step. Cyst ruptures brought a deep internal ache that required prescription painkillers, though I used them sparingly.

Migraines came and went, sometimes stress-induced, sometimes random. No nausea, no swelling, no cramps, small mercies in a body otherwise at war with itself.

There's a strange kind of gratitude that grows in the cracks of pain. I thanked God for what *didn't* happen as much as for what did. I told myself: if this is the worst of it today, I can handle it.

Despite the pain, I pushed on. Fatigue came, but I refused to call it defeat. I traveled, taught, exercised when I could, and worked every day until the transplant.

Even at an eGFR of seven, I was fully operational; no fog, no confusion, just the sharp, stubborn insistence that I was still in control.

I'd look in the mirror and say, "That's not me, that's not my plan, that's not my story. I'm in charge."

Work, Teaching, and the Mask of Normalcy

To outsiders, I looked healthy. I wore suits, spoke confidently, led meetings, and delivered lectures with precision.

Only I knew the quiet choreography it took to get through each day.

Sometimes I'd roll my sleeves down to hide the cotton tape from morning blood draws. Sometimes I'd step out of meetings, out of class, take a deep breath, and remind myself that pain doesn't define presence.

I lived by the Navy creed: ***"Embrace the suck."*** There was no other option.

Work was more than an obligation; it was proof of life. At SAP, Oracle, at Yale, Quinnipiac, The New School, and later at RTX, I built and led with the quiet knowledge that every hour mattered. My students at Quinnipiac and teams gave me something illness couldn't touch: relevance, impact, purpose.

No one knew that between meetings and lectures, I was watching my creatinine climb.

There's a comfort in invisibility when your illness is internal. It allows you to choose when to be vulnerable, when to protect others from your truth. But that invisibility comes at a cost.

You start to forget how to rest.

Moments of Reckoning

The reckoning came in November 2023. I walked into Dr. Chang's office for what I assumed would be another routine visit. We'd been doing this for nearly seventeen years, measure, compare, adjust, repeat (wash, rinse, repeat). But that day, her tone changed.

She looked at the numbers, then at me, and said softly, "We've reached the point. I have to refer you for a transplant."

The room didn't spin, but the air grew heavy. I nodded, said little, and thanked Dr. Chang as I always did. But when I reached my truck, I sat in silence. For the first time in years, the warrior went quiet.

The truth caught up to me: I was done holding the line. This wasn't theory anymore; it was time. I remember gripping the steering wheel, eyes wet, whispering to myself, "This is real. Now what?"

It wasn't fear that followed; it was logistics. How do I tell Marcia? The kids? How do I prepare them for what's next?

That moment became the hinge between acceptance and action. Courage, I realized, isn't loud. Sometimes it's the silent resolve to plan your next move through tears.

Coping and Continuance

Faith filled the spaces where medicine couldn't reach.
I began each morning with a simple prayer: "God, keep me steady."
The words became a rhythm as reliable as breath.

Rituals mattered. Early mornings. Work. Movement. Tracking numbers. My spreadsheets became an extension of myself, columns for potassium, protein, eGFR, and creatinine. Data gave me structure; faith gave me peace. Together, they kept despair in check.

I built redundancy into life the way I did in systems: if Plan A failed, Plan B was ready. If B failed, Plan C stood by. It was how I lived, how I led, how I believed.

My mantra crystallized from years of repetition: **"No guarantees. Do now, not later."** It was equal parts command and confession.

I also borrowed a creed from my Navy days, one that echoed through the halls of those I knew who were SEAL operators: **"The only easy day was yesterday."**

It reminded me that there are no easy days, only the ones we define through discipline and will. We set our own cadence. We choose our own course.

Faith, Family, and Friendship

Marcia stood as my anchor through every unseen storm. Her quiet strength balanced my relentless motion. When I wavered, she steadied. When I refused to stop, she let me move but kept a watchful eye. She knew the difference between allowing me to fight and letting me fall.

Friends like Zac and Jason brought levity when things grew heavy, constant voices of encouragement who never treated me as fragile. And Ryan, my colleague, friend, and eventually my donor, remains a living testament to grace in action. Even before the transplant, his presence was one of reassurance, proof that goodness circulates through the world even when the body falters.

Then there were my students. They saw the professor, not the patient. They didn't know the battle behind the lectures, but their energy and curiosity became medicine of another kind.

A few even asked how they could get tested to be donors. I remember one writing, "Professor, what do we have to do?" I smiled but declined. I couldn't ask that of them. Still, their compassion became a quiet balm, a reminder that humanity is alive and well.

Bridging Survival and Transformation

Somewhere along the way, the narrative shifted. I stopped defining myself by what was failing and started focusing on what was still working. Teaching, leadership, faith, they weren't distractions. They were lifelines.

Purpose became the bridge between survival and transformation. Faith reinforced it. Acceptance sealed it.

I stopped waiting for health to return and began living as though wholeness was already here. That mindset didn't heal the kidneys, but it restored the soul.

I learned that the key to dignity wasn't denial, it was direction. To keep moving forward even when the body wanted to stop.

To lead even when the world said, "Rest." To smile even when the pain pulsed beneath the surface.

When the body betrayed me, I leaned on systems, faith, and people. When fatigue whispered defeat, I countered with belief. And when the future felt uncertain, I planned anyway.

Reflection - Life Inside the Numbers

Living with CKD/PKD isn't just a medical experience; it's a reeducation in humility. A way of life. It teaches patience, endurance, and gratitude, each delivered in doses only life can prescribe.

Living with chronic illness also changes the way you inhabit time. Days stretch and compress in unpredictable ways. Some mornings feel almost weightless, as if, for a brief moment, the body has forgotten its burden. Other mornings feel heavy before you even stand, a quiet signal that the climb will be steeper today. I learned to read my body not just through symptoms, but through subtleties: how quickly I caught my breath on the stairs, how long it took for my muscles to wake, how much resolve I needed to begin.

What surprised me wasn't the inconvenience of illness, but how it rearranged my relationship with time. Minutes I once rushed through became signposts. A quiet sunrise on the way to work. The sound of my kids laughing in another room. The familiar cadence of

Marcia's footsteps in the kitchen. Illness doesn't slow time; it teaches you to slow your life within it.

Every lab draw, every appointment, every test became a meditation on presence. The needles no longer scared me. The numbers still did, but they also guided me. I learned that control isn't about changing outcomes; it's about changing outlooks, meeting each day as it is, not as I wanted it to be.

As the years progressed, I began spending my energy like currency. When your reserves are limited, you spend them deliberately. I worried less about things that once felt urgent but were ultimately meaningless. Purpose became the filter through which I built my days: family, work that mattered, teaching, and faith. Everything else became noise, and I learned to be silent.

But with that clarity sometimes came guilt, guilt for resting, guilt for being tired, guilt for saying "not today." As a veteran and a leader, I was conditioned to push through pain, to keep moving no matter the obstacle. Chronic illness forced me to confront a harder truth: sometimes strength looks like stopping. Sometimes courage means stepping back, not forward. Rest isn't surrender; it's recalibration.

Through it all, a quiet companionship formed between God and, not in dramatic revelations, but in the small, ordinary spaces of my life. Early morning drives to the lab where streetlights blurred like soft halos. Evenings in my office, long after everyone else had gone home. The chapel-like silence of hospital waiting rooms. My prayers were simple: keep me steady, keep them steady, keep us moving.

For nearly two decades, I lived between hospital corridors and boardrooms, between faith and science, between what could fail and what must not. That balance, delicate and deliberate, became the art of endurance.

And in time, the daily grind of CKD became less a burden and more a discipline. Each step, each test, each act of restraint became a kind of devotion, not to disease, but to life itself. The same traits that carried me through deployments and leadership crises carried me through the long waiting season: order, courage, and faith in something larger than myself.

Looking back now, those years were an apprenticeship in endurance. Resilience wasn't forged in dramatic moments; it was built in the ordinary ones, showing up, keeping routines, refusing to let fear narrate the story, choosing hope even when the numbers suggested otherwise. Chronic illness didn't take life from me; it sharpened it. It clarified what matters, deepened who I am, and taught me to walk forward even when the path ahead was dimly lit.

Those years inside the numbers built a foundation stronger than fear: a life anchored in discipline, love, faith, and the quiet, steady courage to keep going.

Chapter 5

Mind Over Matter

There's a saying I've carried for years: "The body listens to the mind, and the mind listens to faith."

Living with a disease like PKD taught me that survival wasn't just a matter of medicine; it was a matter of mentality. The real battleground was never under my ribs; it was between my ears. Mind over matter wasn't a slogan to me; it was a daily operational doctrine. And over time, it evolved into something larger, life over matter.

Faith first, always. Focus next. Then discipline, the hardest of them all. Because discipline is what makes belief actionable.

Early in my journey, I began to shape a personal principle that became a sort of internal compass: **Head EAST, Engage, Adapt, Survive, Thrive**.

It started as a reminder taped above my desk and grew into a mindset I lived by. **Engage** meant showing up every day, even when I didn't want to. **Adapt** meant adjusting course when plans shifted, and they always did. **Surviving** meant holding the line. And **Thrive**; that meant refusing to let PKD define the boundaries of my life.

Over time, another principle joined it, quieter, but just as vital: **be perfectly amenable.** I came to understand that the only true constant in life is inconsistency. Things change. People change. Plans change. The body changes. Accepting that truth didn't weaken me; it steadied me. When you stop fighting the current, you start steering with it. That mindset made the difference between resistance and resilience.

Engage: Faith in Motion

For me, engagement began with faith.

God, family, and country, that order has been my anchor since the Navy. I've worn uniforms, suits, and scars, but my allegiance never wavered. Faith gave meaning to pain, structure to chaos, and patience to uncertainty. It reminded me that not every battle needed to be fought with fists or force. Some were fought through stillness, through trust.

Each morning started the same way: prayer before data. Before I even checked my lab results, I grounded myself in gratitude. I'd whisper a simple prayer, "God, keep me steady today", and breathe deeply until the anxiety in my chest loosened its grip. That was engagement. Showing up for life, even when my body wanted to call in sick.

I learned that every small act, walking, teaching, showing up to meetings, even just smiling, was an act of defiance against despair. Mind over matter didn't mean ignoring pain; it meant overriding fear.

My military background reinforced that truth. In the Navy, we were taught that chaos doesn't wait for permission; you adapt, or you perish. That mindset blended seamlessly with faith. The mission wasn't to win every battle; it was to stay in the fight.

Adapt: The Strategy of Survival

I learned quickly that PKD doesn't care about plans, but I made them anyway.

Having goals written down, visualized, and scheduled gave me clarity when my body gave me noise. I'd write down targets for the week, not just professional tasks, but personal ones too. "Check labs. Drink 3 liters. Read scripture. Thank someone." Simple but intentional.

Some days, my adaptation plan looked like a flight checklist: hydration, blood pressure, diet, work commitments, rest. Other days, it was survival by improvisation; when fatigue hit or a cyst ruptured, I'd pivot, cancel a meeting, reschedule a class, and regroup. Adaptation was not weakness; it was wisdom.

I began practicing small visualization rituals, picturing calm, breathing slowly, seeing pain as temporary data. Over time, gratitude became its own form of meditation. I'd count blessings like I once counted flight hours.

Every small victory, a stable lab, a normal MRI, a clear day without pain, became fuel. I learned that small wins are big wins, and small steps are augmenters of progress.

Each minute became a blessing. Each hour of strength became a reason to thank God.

The result? My mind became trained to see motion, not stagnation, progress, not pause. In the stillness of struggle, there was movement if I chose to see it.

Survive: The Unbreakable Will

There were cracks, of course, moments when fatigue took hold, when the weight of it all pressed hard. I had my share of dark mornings, waiting for lab results, or nights replaying what-ifs in my head.

Fear visited. Anxiety lingered. Anger flared. But I never gave them the keys.

When those moments came, I'd talk myself through it like a commander managing a crisis: Pause. Assess. Reorient. I'd remind myself how far I'd come, seventeen years, countless tests, and still standing.

I had this stubborn Irish streak that refused to yield. Maybe it was heritage. Perhaps it was the Navy. Maybe it was faith. Probably all three. But giving in? Not an option.

Even in moments of frustration, those long waits for labs, or the quiet after Dr. Chang's updates, I told myself: "Look how far you've gotten. You've got this. Forge forward."

I've always believed that the measure of strength isn't how loud you roar, but how quietly you carry.

For me, surrender wasn't the opposite of strength; it was the recognition that I couldn't control everything. I learned to yield when logic or faith demanded it, when I was diagnosed, and when Dr. Chang said it was time for a transplant. Those were moments where I didn't give up; I handed over the reins to God.

Yielding wasn't defeat; it was delegation.
The mission continued, just with new orders.

Thrive: Purpose Beyond Pain

Oddly enough, I never hit what people call "rock bottom." My formation wouldn't allow it. The Navy ingrained in me that pain is information, not identity. PKD became another problem to solve, another mission to execute.

Even at my lowest eGFR, I was still teaching, still leading, still moving. I'd look in the mirror and think: You've still got work to do, fella. Others are counting on you. Get up.

I realized early on that leadership is medicine in its own right. Having others depend on you pulls you beyond self-pity. I couldn't quit, not when students were waiting for class, not when my team needed direction, not when my family depended on stability.

When fatigue hit, I reframed it. "You're tired, but you're still blessed." When fear whispered, I countered. "Faith has the floor."

That mental call-and-response became instinct.

Work and teaching became my proof of life. During difficult periods, job transitions, corporate reductions, moments of uncertainty, I returned to mind over matter as a command phrase. It meant: Stand tall. Lead steady. Keep going.

At times, I thought back to Baghdad, to the days of corkscrew landings and convoy delays, to the discipline of executing under fire. Those experiences had built the same muscle I was using now, not physical, but mental endurance. I'd seen the worst of environments, and I knew: calm is a choice.

That mindset carried me through countless professional storms, layoffs, long nights, complex projects, and even teaching late after full workdays. PKD never got to define me. The mission did.

Authenticity Over Armor

Many people with chronic illness live a dual life, the public mask and the private truth. I never felt that split.

I chose authenticity early. It didn't mean full disclosure to everyone; it meant no duplicity with myself.

I was never ashamed of my condition. It was part of me, but not the defining chapter. I've had an extraordinary life, Navy, DoD, SAP, Oracle, Yale, Quinnipiac, The New School, RTX; teaching, family, and that gave me perspective. There was no need for pretense.

Being real gave me strength. Authenticity disarms fear. It turns vulnerability into authority.

If anything, it deepened my leadership. Teams and students could sense that I understood struggle, even if they didn't know the specifics. Authentic leaders don't need to be perfect; they need to be human.

That truth helped me lead with empathy, patience, and calm, traits I might not have learned without PKD.

The Battle Between Grit and Grace

Mind over matter isn't just about willpower; it's about balance.

Too much grit without grace leads to burnout. Too much grace without grit leads to complacency. I had to learn that both were essential.

Grit kept me moving; grace kept me whole.

There were days when my body felt heavier than armor. Days when even getting dressed took focus. But I never considered myself sick; I considered myself operational.

I wasn't fighting PKD; I was coexisting with it, strategically. I learned to pace, to plan recovery like a mission phase. Fatigue became data, not drama.

And when setbacks came, I leaned on grace, the faith that my life had meaning beyond productivity. That my value wasn't tied to output but to purpose.

In the long arc of this illness, I learned something most people only discover late: strength isn't about control. It's about composition, what you're made of when control is gone.

After Transplant: Gratitude Over Grit

After my transplant, mind over matter took on a new tone, quieter, humbler, more spiritual.

For seventeen years, my mindset had been a shield, and I was fighting on. Now, it has become a lens. Instead of bracing for battle, I began noticing blessings.

I realized that the purpose of mental toughness isn't to block pain, but to channel it into wisdom.

Post-surgery, I was clear-eyed. I saw my duty differently, not just to survive but to honor the gift. Ryan's kidney wasn't a transaction; it was grace in human form. That changes how you think.

I understood that resilience isn't just grit, it's gratitude in motion.

Every sunrise after surgery felt like an answered prayer. My duty was to protect that gift, to ensure my body and mind were strong enough to steward it.

When small obstacles arose, medication side effects, and early fatigue, I returned to the same playbook: engage, adapt, survive, thrive. The framework still worked, only now it was infused with thanksgiving rather than urgency.

Mind over matter had evolved. It was no longer about defying limits; it was about defining purpose.

Lessons in Mental Command

Looking back, I can see that resilience is both a discipline and a decision. It's not innate, it's built.

If I were to teach one lesson to others, patients, caregivers, or healthcare professionals, it would be this: adversity is a universal language. It visits everyone, but not everyone learns to speak it.

The key is to remember three things:
- You are never truly alone.
- You can always act; even small actions count.

- You must never surrender hope, even when logic wavers.

We live in a culture obsessed with control, yet healing often requires surrender. There's wisdom in both.

If you can't control the outcome, control the outlook. If you can't change the pace, change the posture. If you can't stop the storm, adjust the sails.

Resilience isn't a superpower; it's a series of small choices made repeatedly in the face of fear.

When the mind says I can't, faith answers You can.
When the body says Stop, purpose whispers One more step.

That's mind over matter. That's life over matter.

Anchors and Affirmations

Throughout the journey, I kept coming back to a few anchors, mental touchstones that grounded me when life blurred.

The first was my **EAST** principle, Engage. Adapt. Survive. Thrive. Simple enough to remember under stress, yet powerful enough to guide my life.

The second was a mantra I lived by:

- **"No guarantees. Do now, not later."**

One phrase that I live by and still do is:

- **"Tomorrow is only a promise, not a guarantee."**

That phrase became a north star. It reminded me that delay is a thief, and action, even imperfect action, is how you reclaim control.

And finally, scripture became my steady hand. From Galatians 6:9:

"Let us not grow weary in doing good, for at the proper time we will reap a harvest if we do not give up."

Those words hit differently when you've lived through sickness, surgery, and survival. They're not poetic, they're practical. Don't give up, because you can't know how close the harvest truly is.

Mindset as Medicine

If I've learned anything from these years, it's that the brain is the most powerful organ in the body.

Medicine treats, but mindset heals.

I've seen patients with perfect labs crumble under despair, and others with failing organs radiate peace. The difference is where they aim their attention, inward or upward.

For me, mental strength came from believing that life is never static, that even in waiting rooms, something sacred is unfolding.

The human spirit has a strange elasticity. It can bend, twist, even fracture, but it remembers its shape.

And while the body may falter, the mind, guided by faith, can carry the soul across impossible distances.

Reflection - Commanding the Mind

Today, I look back not just as a survivor but as a student of endurance.

Mind over matter was never about ignoring pain; it was about defining perspective.

Every MRI, every blood draw, every lecture taught on low energy, every sleepless night was a lesson in command, not of others, but of self.

That command rests on one truth: the **mind obeys what the heart believes**.

And I believe in faith. I believe in purpose. I think that every hardship has an echo, one that carries forward to strengthen someone else's fight.

For those still navigating their own storms, I'd offer this:
You may not control the diagnosis, but you can control the dialogue within.

When your thoughts spiral, pause and reframe. When your fear shouts, whisper back with belief. When your path narrows, remember, narrow paths often lead to higher ground.

Discipline beats despair.
Faith overcomes fear.

And the mind, anchored in purpose, can move mountains even when the body can't climb them.

Years later, I still live by the same creed: **Head EAST. Engage, Adapt, Survive, Thrive**.

It's not just a principle; it's a prayer in motion.

Because life, like flight, like faith, like recovery, is about heading east toward the light, and when you do, every shadow eventually falls behind you.

III

The Transplant

Chapter 6

Managing the Waiting

The day Dr. Chang told me she was referring me for a transplant didn't arrive with drama or crashing thunder; it came the way truth often does: quietly, firmly, and with no room left for denial.

I had walked into her New Haven office for what I assumed would be another routine evaluation, the kind we had repeated for nearly seventeen years. We reviewed labs, discussed numbers, compared trends, and moved on. PKD had become a steady drumbeat, a background noise I learned to work around. But that day, the rhythm changed.

She looked at the latest labs, then at me, and her expression shifted ever so slightly.

Not fear. Not pity. Just clarity.

"Daniel," she said, "it's time. I'm referring you for a kidney transplant."

Even when you expect these words, they still land like an impact. Expected but unexpected and anticipated but still disarming.

I felt a wave roll through me, not panic, not shock exactly, but a tightening, a recognition that the chapter I had quietly been bracing for was finally here. My throat dried. My mind flooded with questions before I asked them.

Moreover, I did ask them what felt like a thousand.

How bad are the numbers?
What's the timeline?
Will I need dialysis?
Which center?
What do I do next?

She answered everything with the same calm, clinical steadiness she had shown since day one. When she said Yale would be the first referral, I nodded. However, then the strategist in me kicked in.

"Can I also be listed with Hartford Hospital? And the VA? Even other centers?"

She didn't hesitate.

"Yes. In fact, that's better. More centers mean more options."

It was practical advice, delivered plainly, but those words planted the seed of hope I needed. Options meant opportunity. Opportunity meant odds. Furthermore, odds, even slim ones, could be beaten.

The appointment ended, and I carried the weight of her words out the door. When I reached my truck in the parking garage, I climbed in, shut the door, and sat perfectly still for a moment that felt like an eternity.

Then it hit.
The fear.
The reality.
The "What the fuck do I do now?" moment.

I gripped the steering wheel with both hands until my knuckles whitened. I wasn't crying, but the pressure behind my eyes built like a storm threatening to break. For the first time in years, the warrior in me went quiet.

How do I tell Marcia?
How do I tell the kids?
What does this mean?
What if…?

But then, something familiar took over, that mental muscle memory forged through the Navy, hardship, and faith. A shift from emotion to execution.

All right, fella. Engage. Adapt. Survive. Thrive.

By the time I pulled out of the garage, the plan was already forming.

And so began the wait.

A Holding Pattern With No ETA

People imagine waiting for a transplant feels like a countdown, like a clock ticking down to salvation.

But the truth is, it's mostly a holding pattern.

A long one.

Not passive, not idle, but suspended between two worlds: the life you're still living and the life you're waiting to reclaim.

My mind wavered between hope and math. The statistics for Connecticut were sobering:
Five to seven years for a deceased donor.
One to two years for a living donor.
Even the VA projected five to seven years.

I knew the numbers. I knew the odds. I also knew my eGFR was down to **7**.

It doesn't get much closer to the edge than that.

But oddly, I wasn't spiraling. I had spent nearly seventeen years living with PKD; waiting wasn't new, only the stakes had changed.

Still, there were quiet fears I didn't talk about.
What if I never get the call?
What if I die before a kidney comes?
What if dialysis becomes inevitable?
What if I can't finish my doctorate?
What if I can't keep working?

The fear beneath all fears, one I rarely voiced, was shaped by history more than medicine:
My father died at sixty.
My mother died at sixty.
My brother died at fifty-three.

Mortality wasn't theoretical for me. It was familiar.

But every time fear crawled up the walls of my mind, faith answered it. I told myself what I knew to be true: *God has my six.* His timing, not mine.

So I waited, actively, intentionally, and without surrender.

The Logistics of Survival

The waiting period wasn't gentle. It wasn't restful. It wasn't even still. If anything, life sped up.

Within weeks, I was listed at:

Hartford Hospital

Yale New Haven Transplant Center

The VA West Haven Transplant Program

Three centers. Three sets of requirements. Three different rhythms.

Every step mattered. Every appointment mattered. Every lab mattered.

Weekly labs

Vials upon vials to track:

Creatinine

eGFR

BUN

Potassium

Phosphorus

Hemoglobin

Tacrolimus risk baselines

Liver enzymes

Metabolic panels

Parathyroid levels

Sometimes it felt like my veins were a revolving door.

Imaging

CT scans. MRIs. EKGs. Stress tests. Ultrasounds. Cardiology clearance. Vascular mapping. Tests layered on tests.

Diet and hydration

I became almost machine-like in discipline:

3 to 4 liters of water a day

Low sodium

Low phosphorus

Low potassium

1,500 calories per day

Reduced protein

Zero indulgence

I dropped **20 pounds** before transplant.

It wasn't vanity. It was survival.

Fatigue

Oddly enough, I didn't feel "sick." People looked at me and saw a healthy man. But every night, I collapsed into bed like my body was collecting its debt.

Eight to ten hours of sleep.
Every night.
Non-negotiable.

Close calls

In April 2024, dehydration hit hard. Yard work, cutting trees, assembling a gazebo, and stubbornness disguised as productivity. A cold turned into a full ER visit.

Later, after the transplant, the scars intensified, but those would be their own chapters.

During the waiting period, the body was not screaming, but it whispered constantly: *You're running out of time.*

Preparing for Dialysis Without Accepting It

Dialysis hovered over me like a storm cloud.

By every medical standard, I *should* have been on dialysis.

An eGFR of 7 is not survivable for most people without it.

But I was still working two jobs. Still teaching. Still completing my doctorate. Still showing up.

Still fully operational.

Every doctor warned me it was coming.
Every transplant coordinator clarified timelines.
Every nephrology note emphasized "imminent dialysis."

So I prepared for it; mentally, logistically, strategically.

Three days a week.
Early morning sessions.
Get it done, then work, then teach.
Stay alive with structure.

I had my plans.
I had my contingencies.
I was ready.

But I never needed it.

Everyone said it didn't make sense.
I knew the truth: God had bought me time.

Holding the Line at Work

Most people didn't know how sick I was.

To the outside world, I was still:

An executive leader

A CIO driving transformation

An adjunct professor teaching analytics and AI

A father, husband, mentor, protector

Authenticity didn't mean announcing my illness. It meant not lying to myself. So I told the people who needed to know, the CFO, the VP of Finance (who would later become my donor), and a few trusted colleagues.

But to everyone else, I was... normal.
Functional.
Leading.
Delivering.
Stable.

Even when I wasn't.

I hid the fatigue expertly.
The dark circles.

The early morning lab tapes under long sleeves.

The nights of poor sleep.

The mental load.

Teaching helped. It gave me purpose.

Work helped. It gave me discipline.

Faith helped. It gave me peace.

But the wait, the wait tested every role I held.

Especially being a CIO.

We were reducing costs, reducing staff, and still expected to deliver *more* with *less*. It was the wrong season for weakness.

So I didn't allow any.

Leadership became its own kind of medicine. Each problem I solved reminded me that I could still contribute. Still matter. Still lead.

The Private Battle at Home

My family saw more than others, but even then, I shielded them.

Marcia was unshakable, a pillar through every storm. But I knew she was afraid, even when she hid it out of respect for my own peace.

My children understood the stakes, yet they never burdened me with their fear. They supported. They encouraged. They prayed.

My sisters came forward with love and quiet concern. Each had their own fear but kept it behind gentle words.

We talked about risk, openly, honestly, especially between Marcia and me. I had all my affairs in order, including life insurance. Legal documents. Instructions. Not out of pessimism, but out of responsibility.

Yet despite everything, life at home continued. No dramatic disruptions. No collapse of routine. We lived, laughed, argued, cooked, cleaned, and life remained life.

And maybe that normalcy is what saved me.

Faith as Fuel

Throughout the waiting period, my faith sharpened, not softened.

Daily prayers.

Daily conversations with God.

Daily grounding.

Not once did I doubt Him.

Not once did I bargain.

Not once did I feel abandoned.

My entire life, military, academic, and professional, had taught me discipline. But my faith taught me to surrender. Not the giving-up type, but the giving-over type.

God had my six.

Maybe not how I wanted or when I wanted.

But always.

"Slow is smooth. Smooth is fast."

"Hurry up and wait."

Principles from the Navy blended with scriptures and gratitude.

Waiting wasn't passive; it was preparation.

The Mindset of the Unknown

To keep a sense of control during the uncontrollable, I made "what-if" plans constantly. Multiple scenarios. Multiple outcomes. Multiple timelines.

It wasn't anxiety, it was readiness.

Being "perfectly amenable," as I came to call it, meant accepting that life is inconsistent by design. Adaptation became a spiritual exercise, not a tactical one.

And I reminded myself:

I had waited seventeen years to reach the point of being told I needed a transplant. Waiting was not a pause; it *was* the journey.

Time became precious.

Every minute mattered.

Never delay what you can do today.

Tomorrow is a promise, not a guarantee.

The Moment Before the Call

People imagine that the day before the transplant call, you're nervous, pacing, anxious.

Not me.

Truthfully, I was convinced I wouldn't get that call for years.

But being realistic didn't mean being passive. I made it a mission to find a living donor. Dr. Serrano had once told me, "Do everything you can, put up a billboard if you must." The message was clear: be relentless. So I reached out to friends, colleagues, former students, and quiet corners of my life. I even used social media, not dramatically, never with pressure, but with honesty, to share what I was facing and what the road ahead required. It felt strange at first, vulnerable even, but it also felt necessary. If I was going to keep fighting, finding a living donor had to become part of my purpose. I owed that to my family, to my future, to the life I still believed I had left to live.

I went about my normal routines, worked, taught, wrote, and lived.

And then, without warning, everything changed.

Not a false alarm. Not a maybe. Not a "be ready."

A clear, direct message:
You have a donor.

And in that instant, the waiting ended, not quietly, not gently, but with the force of a miracle.

But that moment belongs to the next chapter.

Reflection - Waiting as a Spiritual Discipline

Looking back now, the waiting wasn't wasted time. It taught me the art of steady endurance. It sharpened my faith. It strengthened my roles. It revealed my foundations.

Waiting didn't weaken me; it prepared me.

It showed me that the transplant journey isn't just physical.
It's mental.
It's emotional.
It's spiritual.
It's relational.

It tests every layer of who you are.
But if you approach it with faith, intention, and discipline, the waiting doesn't break you; it builds you.

And by the time the call finally comes, you're not just ready for surgery.

You're ready for renewal.

Chapter 7

The Call That Changed Everything

There are moments in life when time slows, when the air thickens, and the world shrinks to the size of a single sentence. I didn't know it yet, but May 9th, 2024, would become one of those moments, a day I would carry with me the way some people carry medals or scars. It was the day my waiting ended. The day a stranger's voice on the phone spoke words that would alter the course of my life, my health, and my future.

I was in my home office, between Microsoft Teams calls, switching back and forth between my responsibilities as CIO and grading papers for my students at Quinnipiac. It was a Thursday morning, roughly 10:30 a.m. I remember the light coming through the blinds, the quiet hum of my computer, the familiar tension of trying to do three things at once, a typical day in every way except for the undercurrent I had learned to live with: the quiet vigilance of waiting.

The transplant team had told me, "Don't silence your phone. Don't put it on Do Not Disturb. Ever." So when my cell buzzed, I glanced down.

The caller ID read: **Hartford Hospital Transplant.**

My breath caught. My pulse tightened. I answered.

"Hello, this is Dan."

A warm voice, one I recognized, replied, "Hey Dan, it's Andy from the transplant team. How are you doing?"

"I'm good," I said, steadying myself. "What's up, Andy?"

There was a pause. A long one. And in that microscopic quiet, my mind filled a thousand blanks, bad labs, complications, a setback. I braced for impact.

Then Andy exhaled and said the sentence that split my life into a *before* and an *after*:

"Dan, we've got some news for you... We have a donor for you."

For a split second, the world went silent. No MS Teams notifications. No DMs, No emails. No papers to grade. Just that sentence echoing in my mind.

"We have a kidney for you."

I swallowed, my voice barely audible. "Really?"

"Yes," Andy said, warm and certain. "Congratulations."

My heart surged, my hands trembled, and an involuntary tear filled my right eye, the same eye that, months later, would suffer the corneal ulcer that nearly cost me my vision. In that moment, it didn't matter. Nothing did. A miracle had just landed in my lap, in my living room, in my life.

Andy continued, "The surgery will likely be in August or September. The team will reach out with the next steps."

He didn't say who the donor was.
He didn't have to.
Some part of me already suspected.

But I didn't know. Not yet.

When the call ended, I didn't sit. I didn't breathe. I *jumped*. Like a kid told he'd won the lottery. Like a man who'd been holding onto a rope for seventeen years and suddenly felt the tension release. I whispered, "Thank you, God," then said it louder, then said it again.

In that office, the same one where I had graded exams, built technology roadmaps, written emails, and fought fatigue through the long waiting period, I celebrated like a man who had just been given a second life.

I texted Marcia immediately.

"They found a donor."

She was at work at Avon Public Schools. I knew she couldn't respond right away, but I needed to tell her then and there. Some news is too big for timing. Some truths arrive and demand to be spoken out loud.

A few minutes later, she replied.

"Are you serious? Oh my God, Dan."

Her excitement came through the screen. Relief. Joy. Gratitude.

But the deeper conversations would come later that afternoon when she arrived home, when she walked through the front door and hugged me tighter than she had in months.

For now, I just stood alone in my office, heart racing, mind spinning, hands shaking with adrenaline and disbelief. I had waited seventeen years for this moment. I thought it wouldn't come for many more.

But the call had come.

The story was shifting.

The miracle was in motion.

A Gift Hiding in Plain Sight

In the days that followed, the transplant center asked me a question I wasn't expecting.

"Do you know who your donor is?"

It was early May, just a week or so after the initial call. I had a hunch. I had even told Marcia, "I think it might be Ryan." But I wasn't certain. I didn't want to assume something so sacred.

Ryan and I had met in July 2019 when we both started working at Gotham Greens. He was younger than me by fifteen years. Still, we clicked immediately, two leaders with similar philosophies, similar grit, similar commitment to excellence. Over time, we became friends. Trusted colleagues. Brothers in purpose.

When I told him I needed a kidney, he didn't flinch.

"Dude," he said, "you've done so much for others. Let me do this for you, if I can."

I brushed him off at first. "Ryan, no. I can't let you do that."

But he insisted. And quietly, without making a spectacle, without telling the world, without seeking credit, he started the evaluation process. He completed initial testing near his home in New Hope, Pennsylvania, then traveled to Hartford for additional tests in March 2024.

One night that month, we met for drinks in a Hartford bar. We sat for hours. He told me he was going through an evaluation. I thanked him, but tempered my hope. Testing doesn't mean compatibility. Compatibility doesn't mean approval. Approval doesn't mean timing.

At that point, neither of us knew the truth:

He was a perfect match. Almost textbook.
HLA compatibility that rarely happens when the donor and recipient aren't related.

So when the transplant team asked, "Do you know who it is?" I said yes, but my voice carried a mixture of certainty and awe.

"Yes. It's Ryan."
They confirmed it.
"He's your donor."

It felt unreal. Humbling beyond words. I thought back to every conversation, every moment we'd spent talking about leadership, challenges, family, life. I remembered his strength, his calmness, his values.

In that moment, I understood something profound:

Some people talk about sacrifice.

Some people think about sacrifice.

A rare few *become* sacrifices.

Ryan was one of those rare few.

Telling the People Who Needed to Know

That evening, when Marcia came home, we talked in earnest. We stood in the kitchen, the world outside going about its normal routines while ours had just shifted. Her eyes watered with relief.

"Thank God," she whispered. "Thank God."

We told the kids the next day: Kevin, working full-time; Marissa, also working at the school; and Zach, finishing his freshman year at Quinnipiac.

Their reactions were everything a father could hope for: joy, relief, hope, and gratitude. They had carried fears quietly; they never voiced them to me, but I knew. They had watched my labs drop, watched my energy fade, watched me push through life with determination even as my body betrayed me.

To them, this wasn't just a kidney.
It was a reprieve.
A lifeline.
A chance to keep their father healthy, alive, and present.

And it had come much sooner than anyone had expected.

I had prepared myself mentally to wait until 2027. Maybe longer. The median wait in Connecticut was seven years. Even with multiple listings, Hartford Hospital, Yale New Haven, and the VA, the odds were not in my favor.

But Ryan changed everything.

The Countdown Begins

From the moment the call came until surgery, the timeline flew. Nineteen weeks, a blink in medical terms.

I had weekly labs. More imaging. CT scans. MRIs. ECGs. Stress tests. A battery of tests that blurred into one another. I reduced protein. Watched sodium. Drank liters upon liters of water. Lost twenty pounds. Practiced patience. Practiced faith.

There were no complications. No delays. The transplant machine was notoriously slow in many cases, but it ran like a well-oiled system for us. It was surreal.

With work, I arranged my leave. PTO first. FMLA if needed. I prepared my team to run projects without me. Remarkably, I worked up until the day before surgery, and then resumed working part-time from home barely a week after, picking up Oracle ERP tasks and leadership duties again.

For my teaching at Quinnipiac, I prepared every lecture, every video, every assignment. I taught Week 1 of the semester, then handed the torch to my colleagues while I recovered. And two weeks after surgery, I called the program director and asked, "Can I teach by Zoom?" A week later, I returned to campus in person. Nobody expected it. I didn't care. I was back.

But all of that came later.

In the days leading up to surgery, my focus narrowed: hydrate, prepare, pray, stay steady.

Two days before the operation, Ryan and his parents drove from Pennsylvania to Connecticut. We met for dinner, our families together. It was one of those evenings you don't fully appreciate until later, when you realize you were sitting across from the man who would literally save your life in forty-eight hours.

We laughed. We talked. We ate. And inside, I prayed.

"God, protect him. Protect us both. Guide the surgeons. Direct our steps."

The Night Before the Miracle

The night before surgery, I was calm. Calm in a way that felt almost unnatural. But that's the thing about deep faith, it quiets the noise. It softens the unknown.

I lay in bed in Avon, knowing that in less than twelve hours, I would be lying in an operating room while a surgeon placed someone else's kidney inside my body.

I prayed, not just for me, but for Ryan. His health. His recovery. His peace.

I didn't eat much; the renal diet had become second nature. I didn't pack much: sweatpants, shirt, shoes, my iPhone with the Bible app. I didn't need objects. I needed presence.

Did I fear dying?

Somewhat. Yes.

But I also understood something deeper:

If God called me home, then that was His plan.

If God kept me here, then that was His purpose.

Either way, I trusted Him. Completely.

My last thought before sleep was simple:

"God, thank You. You got me this far."

Dawn of a New Life

The morning of September 4th, 2025, arrived quickly. I woke before the sun, took a shower, dressed, and looked at myself in the mirror, a man at the edge of a transformation he had waited seventeen years for.

Marcia drove me to Hartford Hospital. Ryan and his family were already there, but we could not see them until post-surgery. My sister-in-law Teryl came to support us. Marcia and I waited at the pre-op waiting area until it was my turn to be called.

Then the nurses called me back to pre-op.

That room, bright lights, cold air, unfamiliar sounds, will forever be imprinted in my memory. They gave me a gown. Checked my vitals. Inserted IVs. Connected monitors. Drew what felt like a hundred tubes of blood. Then came the nerve block, a strange, warm wave crawling across my abdomen and down my left side.

But through it all, I stayed calm. Focused. Ready.

Warrior mode activated.

Engage.
Adapt.
Survive.
Thrive.

EAST, the principle I'd lived by, became more than a concept. It became oxygen.

I prayed again. For myself. For Ryan. For our families. For the surgeons. For everyone whose hands would play a role in the next few hours.

When the anesthesiologist asked, "Are you ready?"
I nodded.

"Yes, sir. Let's get it done."

My last thought before going under was gratitude. Pure, overwhelming gratitude.

For Ryan.
For my family.
For my faith.
For every miracle God had orchestrated behind the scenes.

And then, in an instant, the world went dark, and a new life began.

Reflection - The Day Heaven Sent a Lifeline

Looking back, the call didn't just change everything; it revealed everything I had already learned:

Waiting is not wasted.

Faith is not theoretical.

Resilience is not optional.

Miracles are not random.

The call didn't just promise a kidney.

It promised more life.

More purpose.

More time with my family.

More opportunities to serve, teach, lead, and love.

It reaffirmed what I had believed all along:

God had my six.

He always did.

He always will.

Some gifts arrive wrapped in paper.

Some arrive wrapped in sacrifice.

Mine arrived wrapped in the heart of a friend, a man courageous enough to step forward and change the course of another man's life.

That is the call that changed everything.

IV

The Second Life

Chapter 8

The Road to Recovery

When people talk about transplant surgery, they focus on the moment in the operating room, the incision, the surgeons, and the clinical choreography that saves a life. But the truth is, the surgery is only half the story. The other half begins the moment you open your eyes, unsure of where you are, uncertain of what has happened, unsure of whether you made it back.

For me, recovery began with a voice calling my name.

I remember surfacing through layers of darkness like a slow ascent from the bottom of a deep ocean. The world was sound first, vision last. Someone said, "Daniel… Daniel, can you hear me?" The voice was calm, steady, clinical. A nurse. My nurse. The person responsible for catching me as I fell out of anesthesia.

I tried to open my eyes, but they were heavy, blurred, useless. Shapes swirled like shadows behind frosted glass. My speech was sluggish, as if someone had packed my mouth with cotton.

"Where am I… Did I make it?"

My words sounded foreign to me, a half-formed echo of myself.

"You're in recovery," she said. "Surgery went well. You did great. Just relax. Your wife will see you soon."

Those words, *surgery went well*, landed before the meaning did. I took a breath, slow and deliberate. Relief washed over me before I fully understood why. Then came the physical awareness: the cool air, the hum of machines, the sharp antiseptic scent, and the unmistakable feeling of something squeezing my legs rhythmically. Only later did I realize they were compression sleeves, inflating and deflating to keep the blood moving.

My body felt foreign, stitched together, heavy, sore, but not in the kind of pain I had feared. More like deep bruising, the internal ache of a body that had been opened and rearranged.

I drifted in and out, coming awake, slipping back under, as nurses moved around me, checking lines, adjusting drips, listening to my chest, speaking in quiet hospital tones that blurred into the background.

Then I heard a familiar voice.
Dr. Serrano.

He appeared beside me like a figure emerging through fog. My vision was still too blurred to make out details, but the cadence of his voice was unmistakable.

"Daniel, everything went superbly well. It took a little longer than expected; we had a delay on the donor side. But you're both out, and the transplant was flawless."

I nodded weakly. It felt like my neck was filled with sand.

Flawless.

The word settled over me like a weighted blanket, grounding me in the moment. I didn't yet know if Ryan was okay. I didn't know his condition, his pain, his outcome. But hearing that *both* of us were out of surgery was enough.

For now.

I slipped back into a half-sleep, rocked by the beeps of monitors and the rhythmic whisper of air vents. Nurses moved in and out, checking vitals, adjusting tubes, murmuring notes to each other. Time became elastic, minutes stretched into hours, and collapsed into seconds.

At some point, I was moved.

I remember motion. The sensation of being wheeled through hallways, lights passing overhead like stars streaking across a night sky. Then the room, my room, on the transplant recovery floor. Dim lights. The soft shuffle of feet. A nurse introduces herself. Another check on my drains and IV lines. Someone is asking about pain. Someone else is adjusting the temperature.

But the moment that lives clearest in my memory was when a nurse said, "Your kidney is working. It started right away."

Working.
Right away.

Those words hit harder than the diagnosis seventeen years earlier. Harder than the pain of ruptured cysts. Harder than the long shadow I had lived under for almost two decades. For the first time in years, I felt something lift. Something that had weighed on me every day, even when I pretended it didn't.

It was like someone had lifted an anvil from my chest.

That night, when I finally had enough clarity to understand what had happened, I whispered two simple words:

"Thank you."

I repeated them like prayer beads:
Thank you, God.
Thank you, Ryan.
Thank you for today.

I couldn't sleep. I was too awake, too grateful, too alive. Around 10 p.m., still buzzing from adrenaline and awe, I grabbed my iPhone and started texting people, taking selfies, sending updates. I couldn't contain the joy. After years of numbers declining, medications increasing, and fatigue deepening, this was the first true upswing.

It felt like resurrection data.

The ICU and Beyond

The ICU was cool, dim, and quiet in the way only an ICU can be, a strange serenity built on the constant presence of machines. Pumps whirred. Monitors beeped. The intercom cut through with occasional announcements. Footsteps pattered softly across polished floors.

I was there about two hours, drifting between consciousness and sleep, my body adjusting to its new reality. I was sore, sore in ways I can't fully describe, but nothing like the pain I expected: just a deep internal heaviness, the weight of healing.

There was no fear. Not the kind that steals breath. Something in me *knew* I was going to be okay.

Maybe it was faith.

Maybe it was instinct.

Maybe it was the presence of something bigger than medicine.

The next milestone came sooner than expected.

On Thursday afternoon, the day after surgery, I asked if I could see Ryan.

One of the doctors smiled and said, "We usually take bets on who visits who first. Donor or recipient."

That made me laugh. Even laughing hurt, but it felt good.

They helped me walk down the hallway to his room. His dad, Jim, was there, sitting quietly, steady, proud. Ryan looked exhausted, pale around the edges, but strong. Stronger than I expected. His surgery had been more profound, more invasive, more painful. Donating a kidney is no small thing.

We stood for a photo, both of us unsteady, both of us changed forever.

I thanked him first. I don't remember exactly what I said; gratitude can be a clumsy language, but I do remember saying, "Slow is smooth, smooth is fast." A Navy saying I live by.

He smiled, nodded, told me I looked good, strong, even. He was surprised I had walked across the floor to see him.

That moment was the first time the enormity of his sacrifice hit me fully. Seeing him, seeing his pain, his courage, it was overwhelming. A mixture of guilt, awe, gratitude, and something deeper, something primal, something that lives beneath words.

He didn't just save my life.
He gave me back to my family.
He gave my kids their father for years to come.
He gave me a second life.

Returning Home

I was released on Sunday, just four days after surgery. Ryan had been discharged on Friday. Marcia drove us home, her hands tight on the wheel, her eyes watching me more than the road.

Pulling into the driveway felt like crossing a finish line.

My son Kevin opened the front door before I even reached it. "Welcome home, Dad," he said.

Just those four words.
Simple.

Steady.

Perfect.

I sat on the sofa and exhaled deeply, one of those exhalations that leaves the body lighter afterward. I didn't feel fragile. I felt grateful, energized, alive.

The family had set up the sleeper sofa downstairs for me, for easier access, no stairs. They had arranged pillows, blankets, water bottles, and medications. It felt like a mission-ready recovery base.

And in some ways, it was.

I moved slowly at first. Slept upright with a pillow wedge. Ate carefully. Measured every step. But inside, my spirit had already begun running.

The Medications and the Discipline

Recovery means medication, lots of it.

High-dose tacrolimus.

CellCept.

Antibacterials.

Anti-rejection drugs.

Stomach protectants.

Supplements.

Pain relievers.

Morning regimen.

Night regimen.

Strict timing.

No missed doses.

Overwhelming at first, yes, but familiar, too.

Systems.

Schedules.

Discipline.

These were things I knew how to master.

I built spreadsheets:

- medication logs

- dosage schedules

- fluid intake

- potassium, sodium, protein

- calories

- blood pressure

- heart rate

- daily weight

- lab values, creatinine, glucose, WBC, electrolytes

Charts. Graphs. Trends.

The whole analyst's toolkit.

Recovery wasn't chaos.

Recovery was data.

And data was something I could control.

Walking Toward Strength

The day after surgery, I walked almost 10,000 steps around the transplant floor.

It surprised the nurses.

It surprised the doctors.

It even surprised me.

Pain wasn't the limiting factor; determination was the engine.

By week one at home, I was walking five miles a day with Marcia.

By week two, seven miles.

By week three, between 15,000 and 20,000 steps a day.

By week four, I was lifting again, lightly at first, then with more purpose.

Fatigue disappeared.

My breathing improved.

My heart rate stabilized.

My blood pressure normalized for the first time in years.

I felt sharper, clearer, more present.

It was like someone flipped the dimmer switch back to full brightness.

My first true "I'm back" moment happened the morning after surgery, standing in that hospital hallway, holding the IV pole, looking at the world with new eyes.

I said it quietly, to myself:
"I'm back."
And I meant it.

The Emotional Breakthrough

The emotional wave didn't hit until that first night. Lying in the dim glow of the recovery room, the realization settled in:

I survived.

There is a moment after major surgery where your mind catches up to your body. Mine arrived like a quiet whisper:

You're still here.

For the first time in years, I cried, not out of fear, but out of overwhelming gratitude. I thought about my parents, my brother Jim, and my sisters Kathleen and Rose. I thought about Marcia, about our kids, about Ryan lying somewhere in another room, enduring pain so that I could live.

I whispered again, "Thank You."

A second life.
A true second life.
Not metaphorical.
Not poetic.

Actual.

Lessons in Return

Recovery taught me more in a few weeks than illness taught me in seventeen years.

Patience – "Slow is smooth, smooth is fast." Healing does not rush; it unfolds.
Gratitude – For every breath, every step, every morning with no pain.
Mortality – Our time is not guaranteed. But our integrity is always ours to defend.
Surrender – Not surrendering the fight, but surrendering the illusion of control, letting God lead.

Discipline – Before surgery, discipline kept me alive. After surgery, discipline helped me heal in record time.

Faith – The anchor. The compass. The constant presence. "We all talk to God." Recovery is where I learned to listen better.

My advice to anyone entering recovery is simple:

Be hopeful.

Trust the professionals.

Do not give up.

Do not give in.

Fight on.

Your life is worth every ounce of effort.

Ryan's Recovery and the Bond Between Us

Ryan's road was more challenging.

Donor surgery is deeper, more invasive, and more painful. He didn't want to stay in the hospital longer than necessary, so those first days were rough. But within weeks, he regained strength.

I checked on him constantly, texts, calls, small updates. When he returned to Connecticut for his one-month post-op appointment, we met again, this time at a local restaurant. He was doing well. Strong. Steady.

Our bond changed after surgery.

He became a brother, not metaphorically, but literally. His DNA runs through my veins. His kidney sits under my ribs, filtering my blood. Our lives, our stories, our families, they are connected forever.

Yet, life is ironic.

In past chapters of my career, milestones like this were often met with shared celebration. This time, life moved quietly forward. There were no announcements or formal acknowledgments, just a simple, private gratitude between the two of us. And in a way, that quite made Ryan's gift feel even more personal, something sacred that didn't need a spotlight.

But we didn't need corporate applause.

What we share lives far beyond any workplace.

Returning to Life

By week three, I taught my first classes again over Zoom.
By week four, I was back on campus.
By three and a half weeks, I was back to full-time work.

I drove again at week four, clinical clearance in hand.

I walked without pain by day three.

I slept comfortably my first night home.

The world looked brighter.

Colors sharper.

No ammonia or metallic taste.

Air sweeter.

Time is more precious.

And sometimes, in quiet moments, like the night after surgery, I whispered the words again:

"I'm still here."

The Night My Eye Caught Fire

Eight months after the transplant, when life was beginning to steady into routine, I learned again how fragile recovery can be.

It happened in late spring of 2025. I had taught a night class at Quinnipiac and drove home exhausted, the kind of tired that seeps into your bones. I had been awake since six that morning, worked a full day at the office, driven an hour to campus, taught for three hours, and then driven back home. By the time I finally walked through the front door, it was close to ten o'clock at night.

I didn't even realize I had fallen asleep with my contacts in.

Around three in the morning, I woke with a burning sensation in my right eye. Not irritation, burning. My eyes were tearing uncontrollably, and every blink felt like sandpaper. Half-asleep, I stumbled to the bathroom, peeled the dried lenses off my eyes, splashed in rewetting drops, and waited for the relief that never came.

By 3:30 a.m., the tearing had worsened. My vision was blurry, the pain sharper, and when I turned on the bathroom light, my eye was bright red and gunked up. Under ordinary circumstances, I might have waited until morning, but I wasn't ordinary anymore. I had a transplant. I was immunosuppressed. Even small infections had the potential to become serious.

I called the transplant center's overnight line.

The nurse listened carefully and then said, "You need to go to the ER. Now."

There was no panic in her voice, but there was urgency.

I got in the truck and drove myself thirty minutes to Hartford Hospital in the middle of the night, the world still and empty around me. Strangely, it felt similar to the drives I used to make to early-morning Navy drills, quiet road, steady mind, no noise except the engine and your own breathing.

They brought me back within minutes. The PA shone a light into my eye, ran diagnostic dye over the cornea, and stepped back with a kind of clinical concern.

"You've got a corneal ulcer," she said. "It's a bad one."

The word *ulcer* hit harder than I expected. Ulcers belong on the skin or stomach lining, not the eyes. But there it was. She prescribed fortified drops and arranged for me to see an ophthalmologist later that morning.

By the time I reached the specialist, the diagnosis was confirmed: a severe corneal ulcer, likely caused by falling asleep in contacts while my eyes went into REM movement against the lenses. The doctor told me plainly, "You're lucky it didn't go deeper. You could've lost vision."

It was sobering.

I had survived PKD, a transplant, years of declining kidney function, yet here was a tiny, microscopic infection capable of undoing so much progress.

It took six weeks of careful medication, follow-ups, and patience, but the eye healed. No permanent damage. Only a small scar on the cornea, a reminder that miracles do not grant invincibility.

I remember leaving the clinic one morning after a checkup, stepping into the sunlight, and thinking:

Even in recovery, life will test you. But God keeps watch even when you sleep.

The Chainsaw and the Grace of God

Just when I thought the turbulence had settled, life reminded me that recovery isn't a straight line, it's a living thing, full of bends, turns, and blind corners.

It was late August 2025, almost a full year post-transplant. I was feeling strong again, teaching, working, writing, moving through my days with a body that finally felt like it belonged to me. My labs were stable. My energy was sharp. My kidney was thriving. For the first time in a long time, I felt... normal.

And then came the chainsaw.

The day started unremarkably. The kind of warm late-summer afternoon that makes the woods feel alive. I was clearing brush and taking down a tall honey locust tree at the edge of my property, a stubborn, dense 60-foot sentinel that had leaned too far into the yard. I had cut hundreds of trees before, over decades. I was careful, methodical, and trained. The Navy had taught me how to plan every angle of a mission, and cutting trees was no different: expect the unexpected.

But sometimes the unexpected still finds you.

As I cut into the trunk, the tree began to twist, not fall, not crack, but twist. Anyone who has cut trees knows that twisting is worse than falling; it's unpredictable, fast, and dangerous. Instinct took over. I pulled my chainsaw back to reposition. My right hand moved to engage the chain brake.

And in the same instant, the tree shifted again.

My hand slipped.

The moving chain met my palm.

I felt nothing at first, not pain, not heat, just impact. A blunt, quick contact, like being struck through a glove. My training kicked in before fear could. I withdrew my hand immediately, finished the cut reflexively, and only when I stepped toward the lawn did I look down.

Blood.

Across my palm, down my fingers. Two long, deep gashes, three to four inches each, running across the base of my hand and into my pinky and ring finger. It looked worse than it felt, which somehow made it more surreal.

I shut the chainsaw off and walked toward the yard where my wife was watering plants. The moment she saw my hand, her face changed, fear and urgency surfacing instantly.

"Just get me the hose," I said calmly. "And some paper towels. Gauze, if we have it."

She hurried inside while I rinsed the blood off under the cold water. My hand still worked, fingers moved, grip intact. No numbness. No loss of function. That alone was a miracle.

When she returned with paper towels and gauze, I cleaned the wounds, applied pressure, and wrapped them tightly. Only then did I allow myself to acknowledge what had just happened. A chainsaw. An immunosuppressed body. A deep cut. And yet... full function. No shock. No panic. Just clarity.

"Let's go to Hartford Hospital," I told her.

She insisted on coming, even as she rushed to get changed. While she got ready, I put the chainsaw away in the garage, climbed into my truck, and waited quietly, hand wrapped, bleeding slowed, mind steady. I wasn't thinking about pain; I was thinking about infection, tendons, bone, and the fact that I was just shy of a year post-transplant. I knew the stakes.

The drive to the ER was familiar, almost routine, another chapter in a medical life that had stretched nearly two decades. They took me in quickly. X-rays were done. Vitals checked. Wound examinations, neuro tests, mobility assessments.

The doctor finally came in and looked at my hand, eyebrows raised.

"Are you sure this was a chainsaw?" he asked, half-laughing. "This looks like a knife wound."

"It was definitely a chainsaw."

He shook his head. "Then you're the luckiest man I've seen this week."

No tendon damage. No bone involvement. No severed nerves. No infection. Just deep lacerations requiring stitches.

When he finished suturing the wounds, he wrapped my hand gently and said, "You're good to go."

And that was it.

Walking back to the truck, hand bandaged, wife beside me, I felt the weight of what could have happened. Not just the physical risk, but the risk to the transplant, the possibility of infection, the fragility of everything I had fought for. A year earlier, my body was on the edge of renal failure. Now it was carrying a miracle inside it, and I was walking out of an ER after a near-miss that could have changed everything.

But it didn't.

Again, God had my six.

I remember sitting in the truck afterward, looking at my wrapped hand, thinking: How many times can one man be carried through? How many times can grace intervene before you admit that you're not lucky, you're protected?

The chainsaw incident didn't scare me. It humbled me. It brought a new kind of awareness, a sharper gratitude for the ordinary moments, holding a cup of coffee, typing an email, teaching a class, gripping a steering wheel. Things I once took for granted became sacred in their simplicity.

In those stitches, I saw a reminder:

Recovery isn't immunity.
Healing isn't invincibility.

Miracles don't end when the surgery is over.

They continue, in the quiet, in the mundane, in the unexpected moments where life could break you, but doesn't.

I walked into the ER with two deep lacerations. I walked out with my hand intact, my body stable, and a renewed understanding that my second chance wasn't just surviving.

It was being protected, guided, held.

And I was, without question, one lucky son of a bitch.

Reflection – From Survival to Strength

Recovery taught me that healing is rarely a straight line; it is a mosaic of gratitude, discipline, and unexpected grace. The first hours after surgery were a blur of machines, voices, sensations, and relief, but beneath the clinical environment was something more profound. A quiet knowing. A sense that God had pulled me through the darkest valley and set me on a path I was never promised but was gifted anyway.

Those early days revealed something I hadn't felt in years: the unmistakable spark of life returning. Not suddenly, not dramatically, but steadily, with each step in the hallway, each prayer whispered in the dark, each moment of seeing my donor and realizing the depth of his sacrifice. Recovery became more than a medical process; it became a spiritual awakening. A reminder that the body can be rebuilt, the mind can be revived, and the soul can be re-centered when grace meets perseverance.

Fourteen months later, the numbers told the story just as clearly as my memories:
eGFR around 92.
Creatinine normal.
Blood pressure is normal.
Heart rate is normal.
Electrolytes stable.
WBC balanced.
Body strong at six-foot-two, 210 pounds, with a 32-inch waist.
Healthy. Alive. Present.

These weren't just lab values; they were proof that the impossible had bowed to faith, discipline, and providence. Proof that a life once defined by decline could rise into strength again. I became living evidence that miracles still happen, that grace still moves, and that sometimes the quietest wars, fought in hospital rooms, ICU corridors, data sheets, prayers, and sleepless nights, lead to the loudest victories. And in those victories, I found not just recovery, but renewal.

Chapter 9

A Better Than Expected Recovery

The first morning home felt like stepping into a different lifetime.

Not just another day, but a new beginning, wearing the clothes of an ordinary sunrise. The light came softly through the living room windows, settling across the pillows and blankets my family had arranged for my recovery space. Five days earlier, I had been on an operating table with a failing organ, years of decline behind me, uncertainty in front of me. Now I stood in my own home, alive and steady, feeling more energy in my bones than I had felt in years.

I woke before the house stirred, habit, discipline, and excitement blending. My mind was clear. My lungs felt fuller. My body felt renewed. There was soreness, yes, the deep kind of soreness that reminds you something extraordinary has happened beneath the skin. Nevertheless, layered over that soreness was something else: joy. Relief. Gratitude.

I remember sitting upright, gathering my new morning medications, lining them up with precision, as if each pill were a symbol of the second chance now beating beneath my ribs.

Furthermore, I felt something I hadn't felt in a long time: purpose. Real purpose. The kind that lifts you from bed before the alarm and makes you grateful for breath itself.

Something inside me knew:
You're healing faster than expected.

And I was.

The Surge of Life

The signs showed up immediately, far earlier than typical post-transplant patterns. The night of the surgery, my new kidney began working almost instantly, producing urine within hours, a rare and reassuring signal that the graft had taken. By the next morning, my eGFR was 65, a number most people don't see until days or weeks into recovery. By the time I was discharged, I was hovering near 80.

Doctors, nurses, techs, and everyone who stepped into my room said the same thing:

"You're doing unbelievably well."
"This is exceptional progress."
"You're recovering faster than expected."

They weren't exaggerating.

Surgery had been on a Wednesday. By Thursday night, I was already walking laps around the transplant floor. Eight, ten, sometimes twelve laps. Enough that nurses would laugh as I passed their station: "You again? You're putting the rest of us to shame."

But the surge, the real surge, hit me the morning after surgery. It was like someone had plugged me into a power source I didn't know existed. A clarity and vitality I hadn't felt since my thirties pulsed through me.

Even now, I remember thinking:
Is this what healthy feels like? I forgot.

First Week Victories

The first week was a series of small victories that felt monumental.

Standing up without help. Walking unassisted to the bathroom the very next day. Showering with a tech on standby, but never needing him. Tying my own shoes, carefully but confidently. Going up and down stairs by day three. Transitioning from a hospital gown to regular clothes. Sleeping deeply through the night, something I had not done in years. Stepping outside once home and walking nearly a mile.

Independence returned in fragments, each one a quiet triumph.

I would catch myself smiling at the simplest things, being able to stand at the kitchen counter, being able to bend slightly without exhaustion, and being able to walk without that familiar sensation of heaviness in my body. These were more than tasks. They were confirmations.

The old me had not disappeared.
He had simply been waiting.

A Family Recentered

Recovery wasn't solitary. It pulled my family closer in unexpected ways.

Marcia was steady and supportive, nervous at times, protective when she thought I was pushing too fast, but she also knew my drive. She knew I was the type who would reassure her even when I had every right to be the one comforted.

My daughter called daily, checked on me, visited, and brought me the kind of tenderness only a daughter can give her father.

Kevin, living at home, was attentive, fetching what I needed before I even asked, carrying things, checking in, offering the quiet support of someone who wants his father to get better.

Zach, away at college but only an hour from home, visited on weekends, called often, texted late-night messages: "Dad, how are you feeling?" "Need anything?"

One moment stands above the rest.

The second weekend at home, all of them were there. The house felt full. They sat around me, talking, laughing, making sure I was comfortable, telling me how good I looked, how strong I seemed.

It wasn't their words that moved me.
It was their presence.

That afternoon, I realized something profound:
My recovery wasn't just mine. It was theirs, too.

Strength Returning Faster Than Science Predicted

I was shocked by how rapidly my physical strength returned. By the end of the second week, I could walk several miles a day. Within weeks, with the doctor's permission, I was exercising again, weights, pushups, sit-ups, the exercise bike, regaining muscle I thought had been lost forever.

Doctors were surprised. Nurses were surprised.

Even I was surprised.

Dr. Serrano smiled every time he saw my labs.

"Remarkable," he said.
"You're healing as if your body has been waiting for this."

Dr. Singh, who managed my longer-term care, was equally affirming. Nurses would lean in when checking vitals: "You look amazing." "These numbers… we don't see this often."

But the truth is, I felt it long before anyone said it.

The surge was real.
The lights were back on.
The engine inside me had restarted.

The Mind Awakens

After the transplant, fear vanished.

Before surgery, yes, the fear was there, fear of complications, fear of disease progression, fear of time running out. But afterward? Recovery felt like faith made tangible. A new organ working inside me, a gift alive and functioning, erased the old anxieties.

In their place came clarity. Determination. Gratitude.

Faith played an essential role. Recovery became a conversation between God and, steady, honest, intimate. In the hospital, I felt spiritual peace settle over me like a blanket. At home, it deepened. There were moments of calm so profound they felt like whispers from something greater.

This transplant wasn't just medical.
It was sacred.

Routine as Redemption

My discipline became a lifeline.

Medications on schedule, precise, timed, consistent. Logs in my spreadsheet: eGFR, creatinine, fluid intake, fluid output, blood pressure, weight, glucose, sodium, protein, and calories. Charts and graphs, trends over time. Patterns I could analyze, understand, and trust.

If surgery gave me a new kidney,
discipline protected it.

Tracking wasn't just data.

It was empowerment.

It was control.

It was foresight.

It was life lived with awareness.

Returning to Teaching, A Different Kind of Healing

By week three, I was teaching again via Zoom.

Week four, I returned to campus.

Students' faces lit up when I appeared at the front of the room. Their shock, their joy, their encouragement, it was all fuel for my spirit.

Some said I looked healthier than before the transplant.

Some said I inspired them.

Some said, "Welcome back, Professor."

Students who had graduated reached out on LinkedIn, by text, by email. Their support was powerful, unexpected yet deeply affirming.

Teaching grounded me.

It stabilized me.

It reminded me why I fight to stay alive with purpose.

Returning to Work, Too Soon, Too Fast

My job, unlike my students, did not send a card.

Did not send encouragement.

Did not send acknowledgment.

Instead, the calls started early.

The asks started early.

The expectations returned before I had even regained full mobility.

Within two weeks, I was working part-time. By week three, full-time. I was supposed to be out six to eight weeks.

But the pressure was relentless.

In hindsight, I should have waited. I should have allowed myself to heal. But determination, pride, and responsibility tugged me back sooner than I should have gone.

Still, every time I looked in the mirror, I said quietly:
"I'm back."

And part of me was right.

Moments of Reflection and Realization

Recovery carried emotional depth, even without tears. Gratitude became my steady companion, a lens through which I saw the past, present, and future.

The day before the transplant and the morning of the surgery remained sharp in my memory, those moments when the possibility of finality hovered close. Drafting my will, preparing my affairs, realizing how fragile everything truly was.

Ryan's sacrifice weighed on me, not with guilt rooted in shame, but guilt rooted in awe.

He had given me life at a cost no one can ever repay.

Every call to check on him, every update, every moment of slow healing on his side reminded me that his generosity was immense.

A gift of that magnitude shapes a man.

It transforms him from the inside out.

Shifts in Identity

The transplant changed the way I viewed work, life, and purpose.

Career?
A career is a tool, not a life.

Health?
One chance. One body. One path.

Family?
A responsibility and a privilege, not to be taken for granted.

Purpose?
Reaffirmed:
Help others. Serve. Teach. Give more than you take.

Time?
Precious. Limited.
Gone before you realize it if you don't guard it.

This wasn't a "second life."
This was a renewed life, purposeful, intentional, grounded.

Fourteen months after the transplant, that renewed sense of purpose carried me somewhere I never expected I would reach so soon: across a graduation stage, completing my Doctorate in Education. Finishing a doctorate less than a year and a half after major surgery wasn't ambition; it was gratitude in motion. It was my way of honoring the gift I'd been given. I wrote papers during recovery, attended classes between lab draws, and pushed through fatigue with the same discipline that kept me alive through the hardest years of PKD. That degree became a symbol of more than academic achievement; it was living proof that my new kidney didn't just restore my health, it restored my momentum, my calling, and my belief that God had more work for me to do.

Foreshadowing What Came Next

By September and October of 2024, I felt myself entirely again, stronger, sharper, more energetic than I had been in decades.

Physically capable. Mentally alert. Spiritually anchored. Determined to reclaim everyday life.

What I did not realize yet was that recovery—even extraordinary recovery doesn't make you invincible. It gives you strength, but strength still needs wisdom. It gives you clarity, but clarity still requires caution.

And life would soon test that knowledge in ways I could never have predicted.

The Message of Recovery

If a specific message resonated from all of this, I would say it is the following:

Believe in yourself.
Trust your medical team.
Have a plan.
Follow the plan.
Reach out to others.
Lean on faith.
Trust in the LORD.
You are stronger than you think.

My recovery was better than expected because I believed, prepared, disciplined myself, fought with purpose, and surrendered with faith.

It was hopeful.
It was triumphant.
It was humble.
It was spiritual.
It was reflective.

It was proof that life can rise from the shadows stronger than before.

Reflection – A Recovery That Reawakened Purpose

Recovery wasn't only a process of restoring the body; it became a process of restoring the soul. As the first weeks passed, I realized the true miracle wasn't just that my kidney began working; it was that my entire life began to sharpen around a more profound sense of calling. Strength returned to my muscles, clarity returned to my mind, and gratitude returned to my heart, each one unfolding like layers of light after a long night.

What surprised me most wasn't how quickly I healed, but how completely I felt reawakened. Every walk, every prayer, every moment with my family felt intentional, deliberate, almost sacred. I didn't think of it as living a second life; I thought of it as living my truest one, anchored by faith, guided by discipline, and fueled by a determination to honor the gift I had been given. In the quiet of early mornings or the stillness of late nights, I found myself whispering thanks, not out of habit, but out of recognition: healing had given back more than health. It had given back purpose.

Moreover, as I stepped into the months ahead, I understood something essential. My recovery was not a finish line or a victory lap; it was a covenant. A promise to God, to my family, to Ryan, and to myself to live with intention, humility, and grace. Whatever came next, teaching, working, serving, walking through the woods with new strength, I carried forward the awareness that life is not guaranteed, but it is entrusted; furthermore, that made every breath feel like both a responsibility and a blessing.

V

The Wisdom Gained

Chapter 10

What I Learned About Resilience

For much of my life, resilience was a word I believed I already understood. It meant showing up, performing, executing—regardless of pain, fear, or cost. It meant strength without sound, stamina without complaint, and discipline without deviation. It meant being the one people could rely on, the one who didn't flinch, the one who didn't break. But living through PKD, navigating seventeen years of uncertainty, accepting a transplant, and rebuilding my life afterward taught me something far more profound: resilience is not measured in what you withstand silently, but in how you accept help, embrace vulnerability, and align strength with purpose. This chapter is about how that understanding evolved. How resilience changed shape, changed meaning, and ultimately changed me.

Before PKD – The Armor of Strength

Before PKD ever disrupted my rhythm, resilience was a professional currency. In the Navy, it meant being operationally ready regardless of circumstance. On executive teams, it meant absorbing pressure so others didn't have to. In the cockpit, resilience was procedural: follow the checklist, trust the instruments, suppress emotion. I thought resilience meant holding the line, not asking for support, and keeping my internal storms hidden behind a steady exterior.

Looking back, I now understand that what I once called resilience was often just survival dressed in discipline. In those years, my definition of resilience was shaped by structure, hierarchy, and mission. It was shaped by an unspoken belief that vulnerability was a distraction and emotion a liability. I learned to compartmentalize, to push forward, to keep moving. And in many moments, career milestones, difficult family seasons, and leadership roles, I believed that enduring silently was noble.

But that definition had limits. It worked in the Navy. It worked in the boardroom. It worked in the classroom. It didn't work against a disease that couldn't be outperformed, outmaneuvered, or outrun.

The Long PKD Years – When Resilience Shifted

Around 2012, PKD began to shift the meaning of resilience from physical to mental. No longer could I simply "push through" fatigue, pain, or declining kidney function. The Navy-like instinct to compartmentalize couldn't fix an illness that moved quietly, slowly, without regard for willpower.

The hardest part of PKD was not pain. It wasn't the fatigue. It wasn't the medication. It was the slow erosion of control. As a leader, a pilot, and a systems thinker, I was used to solving problems. PKD offered no solutions, only management, patience, and surrender.

At work, resilience took a new form. I taught full course loads, led strategic initiatives, advised executives, and built teams, all while running on diminishing internal capacity. I hid symptoms not out of shame, but out of duty. I believed that protecting the system meant protecting others from my illness. I absorbed the emotional tax so others didn't have to.

There were moments of profound weakness that I shared with no one, the nights when kidney pain kept me awake, the heavy guilt when I missed family events, the quiet frustration when lab values dropped despite my discipline. I carried those moments privately because I believed leadership demanded silence.

But slowly, I learned that resilience wasn't about concealment. It was about connection. It was about acknowledging fear without being ruled by it. It was about recalibrating expectations. It was about protecting dignity while the body betrayed instinct.

Marcia played a profound role in this shift. Where I leaned into discipline, she leaned into empathy. Where I suppressed emotion, she let hers surface. She didn't ask me to be indestructible; she asked me to be present. My children gave me a different form of purpose: a reason to keep moving even when hope felt thin. And my faith reframed the journey altogether. PKD wasn't a punishment; it was preparation, an unexpected apprenticeship in humility, perspective, and trust.

Resilience, during these long years, became quieter, deeper, and more relational.

Learning to Accept Help – The Hardest Lesson

I spent decades being the one others relied on. I led teams. I taught students. I mentored colleagues. I carried responsibilities with a sense of duty forged by service. But PKD forced a truth I never wanted to confront: resilience sometimes requires accepting help.

Accepting help felt like surrender. Not because I was prideful, but because I was programmed to lead. The idea of being dependent rubbed against every instinct I had cultivated. But in illness, leadership had to make room for vulnerability.

Ryan's offer to donate a kidney changed everything I thought I knew about strength. He didn't approach it as charity. He approached it as a covenant. A calling. A mission. He embodied a form of resilience I had never fully understood, one built on sacrificial generosity, not personal endurance.

Depending on him for my life was both terrifying and sacred. It forced me to relinquish control, but it also allowed me to experience humanity at its highest expression. His decision redefined strength—not as self-sufficiency, but as selflessness. I learned that vulnerability is not a breach of resilience; it is proof of it.

I also learned that receiving help is its own courageous act. It requires trust. It requires humility. It requires the belief that you are worthy of care. And in those months leading to surgery, I finally understood that resilience is not a solo journey. It's shared.

The Operating Room – Resilience as Surrender

The moments before surgery were strangely calm. I had expected fear, but what came instead was stillness. I prayed, not for outcomes, but for peace. I told myself quietly, "Whatever happens, I'm ready." It wasn't a resignation. It was release.

For seventeen years, I lived with PKD. I led through its symptoms, taught through its fatigue, and carried the quiet weight of uncertainty across continents, classrooms, boardrooms, and ER hallways. If this surgery ended the journey, I had lived well. If it began a new chapter, I was prepared.

In the hours after surgery, resilience took a form I never imagined: surrender. Tubes, monitors, weakness, I couldn't lead, couldn't problem-solve, couldn't perform. But I could breathe. I could trust. I could receive. I let the nurses work, let Marcia anchor me, and let Ryan's kidney begin its quiet miracle.

The moment I realized the kidney was working was holy. The numbers rose. The warmth returned. Relief washed through me. I cried, not out of fear, but out of awe. My identity shifted from executor to steward. Resilience became a sacred responsibility, not a professional tool.

Discipline – The Resilience of Routine

In recovery, discipline wasn't about control; it was about covenant. Logging numbers, tracking medication, walking hallways, monitoring labs, each act was a promise to honor Ryan's gift, Marcia's support, my children's hope, and God's grace.

The spreadsheet became more than data. It became a journal of recovery. A cockpit dashboard in an aircraft, I was learning to fly post-transplant. Every entry was a small victory. Every graph was a prayer in code.

But discipline also became armor. It gave me structure in a season where unpredictability reigned. When fear crept in, fear of rejection, infection, complications, I returned to the spreadsheet. Not as avoidance, but as adaptation. Discipline allowed me to metabolize fear into action.

Resilience wasn't loud. It wasn't dramatic. It was deliberate. It lived in the small acts repeated with purpose.

The Quiet Battles of Recovery

Recovery wasn't linear. The eye ulcer was a jarring reminder that healing has detours. Just when I felt rejuvenated, labs improving, energy rising, the ulcer struck. Pain, sensitivity, disruption. But PKD had prepared me for ambiguity. I responded with precision: triage, ER, follow-up, adaptation. It was another battle, but I had the tools.

Emotionally, recovery surprised me. I expected exhaustion. Instead, I found joy, simple, immediate, profound. I laughed more. I prayed with gratitude, not desperation. It felt like the system rebooted not just physically, but spiritually.

Mentally, the hardest shift was relinquishing the instinct to command. Healing required surrender. It required trust in the kidney, the process, the body, the grace that carried me. I had to loosen my grip on control and embrace presence instead of performance.

Resilience during recovery often meant resting, pausing, or being gentle with myself. Those acts were not retreats; they were recalibrations.

Unexpected Tests – The Eye and the Chainsaw

The corneal ulcer tested my resilience as an immunosuppressed patient in ways the transplant didn't. It forced vigilance, urgency, and humility. In the ER, I wasn't a leader or a professor; I was a patient. Vulnerable, dependent, exposed. But I learned that vulnerability invites care. The ER team responded with urgency and skill. I didn't need to perform strength; I needed to receive it.

The chainsaw accident was another unexpected test. A momentary slip, a flash of danger, and everything could have changed. My instincts kicked in: stabilize, assess, seek care. It reminded me that health is fragile, but resilience is reflexive. Gratitude flooded in, not just for survival, but for the grace woven into every narrow escape.

Both events recalibrated my understanding of recovery. "Recovered" didn't mean immunity from setbacks; it meant readiness to adapt. These moments didn't weaken me; they deepened my faith, sharpened my humility, and reinforced the sense of protection that had hovered over my journey.

Work, Teaching, and Purpose Reborn

Returning to work so soon after transplant, three weeks instead of the recommended six to eight, was a mixture of resilience and obligation. Teaching felt restorative, aligned with purpose. It allowed me to show up authentically, even while healing. Students didn't need perfection; they required presence.

But returning to my executive role felt different. The demands were relentless. There was no margin, no compassion, no acknowledgment of human cost. It wasn't resilience, it was sacrifice. That experience reshaped how I lead today: with empathy, with margin, with respect for human fragility.

A student once told me, "You taught us more by showing up than by anything in the syllabus." That moment crystallized a truth: resilience teaches even when you don't intend it to.

Illness didn't weaken my leadership; it refined it. It stripped away illusion and left clarity: systems must honor humanity, not just output.

Faith – The Core of Resilience

As PKD progressed, prayer transformed. It moved from asking for outcomes to seeking presence. It became quieter, deeper, more relational. I stopped praying as a strategist and started praying as a son. I prayed not to avoid storms, but to anchor within them.

In the operating room, just before anesthesia, I felt God's presence more vividly than ever before. It wasn't silence, it was stillness with a pulse. A knowing that I was held.

Scripture sustained me:
"Bestill, and know that I am God."
"They that wait upon the Lord shall renew their strength…"

Faith was no longer a theory; it was a lived experience. It carried me through lab results, through setbacks, through every quiet battle of body and spirit.

The Lessons Resilience Taught Me

If someone newly diagnosed with PKD asked me about resilience, I would tell them this:

Resilience is not endurance. It is alignment. It is the integration of hope, discipline, faith, and purpose. It is choosing how to live, even when you cannot choose what happens.

To someone waiting for a transplant, I would say:

Prepare your body, but also prepare your soul. The call will come. And when it does, you will not just survive, you will rise.

To caregivers:

Your presence is part of the healing. You sustain the journey in ways medicine cannot measure.

To my children:

Resilience is not about being invincible. It is about being intentional, open, humble, and present. Strength includes vulnerability. Leadership includes rest. Faith includes uncertainty.

The big battles matter. But the quiet ones shape you.

Reflection – The Alignment of Strength and Grace

Resilience, I have learned, is not the capacity to endure endlessly. It is the willingness to align strength with grace. It is the quiet decision, repeated daily, to show up with purpose even when the outcome is uncertain. It is the discipline of hope, the courage of vulnerability, and the humility of trust.

Resilience is not what kept me alive. It is what made life worth living.

And if my story leaves one imprint, let it be this:
You do not carry resilience alone.
You carry it with others, with God, with family, with community, with the unseen grace that meets you in every quiet battle.

Chapter 11

Tips and Best Practices

Resilience isn't abstract to me anymore.

For years, it sounded like a buzzword people attached to military service, leadership roles, or battle-tested careers. "You're so resilient," they'd say when they heard the abbreviated version of my story: Navy, SAP, Oracle, Yale, Quinnipiac, The New School, RTX, CIO, transplant. It sounded flattering. It also sounded distant, like they were describing a concept instead of a life.

But you don't really understand resilience until your own biology turns against you and you still have to show up, for your family, your work, your students, your faith, and yourself.

This chapter is the closest thing I can offer to a field manual.

It's not medical advice. It's lived advice. It's the set of practices, habits, and quiet decisions that helped carry me from diagnosis to transplant and into this strange, sacred second life. If there's a theme that ties it all together, it's this:

Resilience is not one big moment. It's a thousand small choices, made on days when no one is watching.

Medical & Health Practices

The practical things that saved my life.

If I could sit across from my 2007 self, the guy who had just heard the words, "You have Polycystic Kidney Disease. There's no treatment. No cure.", I wouldn't start with comfort.

I'd start with clarity.

I'd tell him, "Start treating your kidneys as if they've already begun failing, because they have."

Back then, I still believed in the quiet myth of invincibility. I was flying, leading, consulting, and building a career. I was used to solving problems with force: more effort, more hours, more grit. PKD doesn't respond to that kind of thinking.

Suppose I had understood that sooner, I would've gotten quarterly labs, not yearly. I would've tracked creatinine the way most people track their checking account. I would've learned what eGFR meant right away and taken every slight fluctuation seriously. And I would've understood that a body under constant stress, dehydrated, sleep-deprived, and overworked—pays the bill eventually, with interest.

Over time, a few daily habits became the scaffolding that held me up as my kidney function slid from the 40s to the 30s, and eventually into single digits:

Hydration first, before anything else. Not after coffee, not "later in the day", first.

Blood pressure every day. On the worst stretches, twice a day. Numbers don't care how "busy" you are.

Low sodium on purpose. Even before I had "official" restrictions, I started reading labels and respecting the impact of salt.

Walking instead of proving something. Not marathons, not gym heroics, just consistent movement.

Sleep as a prescription: same bedtime, same rhythm, and no more treating rest like a luxury.

I logged labs and vitals obsessively, first in notebooks, then in spreadsheets and apps. That logging became my radar. It showed trend lines that emotion would've tried to ignore.

Three lab values became my holy trinity:

Creatinine, the number that never lies.

eGFR, the actual slope of the mountain I was climbing.

The protein/creatinine ratio is the early warning alarm that things are under strain.

When those numbers shifted, my behavior followed: more water, stricter diet, less stress, and a call to my nephrologist. Tracking labs wasn't passive; it was how I made decisions.

Hydration, especially, became non-negotiable. I adopted a crude but effective rule: never let your urine turn dark yellow. Later, I translated that into 65–80 ounces a day, adjusted for heat and activity. Hydration became the daily shield, softening the blow of everything else: long days, travel, illness, and even stacked medications.

Diet shifted from "I should probably eat better" to a strategy:
- Less sodium, because hypertension is PKD's accelerant.
- Moderate protein, not bodybuilding levels, just enough.
- Thoughtful potassium, guided by labs, not fear.
- Less processed food, because phosphorus and hidden sodium are quiet saboteurs.
- Enough calories to stay functional, not starving myself into worse labs.

My biggest mistake early on was simple: because I felt fine, I assumed I was fine.

I waited too long between nephrology appointments. I swapped water for coffee. I underestimated how much sleep and stress were intertwined with blood pressure. I thought discipline could outwork disease.

It couldn't. But once I started respecting sleep, managing stress intentionally, walking daily, avoiding NSAIDs completely, and treating medication timing like a cockpit checklist, we slowed the descent.

If you're living with PKD, three health non-negotiables stand out from my story:

1. Protect your blood pressure as if your life depends on it, because it does.
2. Hydrate more than you think you need, consistently.
3. Never skip labs or nephrology follow-ups.

If there's a fourth: do not touch NSAIDs. That lesson came late for me. I wish it hadn't.

And I wish, very early in my journey, someone had looked me in the eye and said:

"You can't stop PKD. But you can slow it dramatically. You have more control than you think."

That one sentence could have changed everything.

Navigating the System Without Being Crushed by It

PKD is a medical condition. A transplant is a medical intervention. But everything in between is administrative warfare.

By the time I was listed at **Hartford Hospital, Yale New Haven**, and the **VA**, I had learned a hard truth: you cannot passively move through a transplant system and expect it to carry you.

Getting listed at multiple centers is not "gaming the system." It's survival.

Each center has its own philosophy, risk appetite, wait times, and criteria. What one center quietly labels "borderline," another may see as acceptable. Yale, Hartford, and the VA all evaluated me through slightly different lenses. That variation mattered.

But the centers do not manage one another. They do not synchronize. They do not automatically share your story.

You are the connective tissue.

I built what became my "transplant binder", part military flight manual, part CIO playbook. Inside, I kept:

- All lab results, chronologically ordered

- Imaging reports (CT, MRI, ultrasounds)
- A current medication list with dates of changes
- Blood pressure logs
- Insurance cards and authorization notices
- Contacts for transplant coordinators, nephrologists, cardiologists
- Notes from every appointment
- A timeline of major events and symptoms

That binder changed the tone of every encounter. When someone asked, "When did your creatinine jump?" I had the date. When insurance challenged coverage, I had the paper trail. When a new specialist needed to understand seventeen years in fifteen minutes, I had the map.

Advocacy is not aggression. It's clarity plus persistence.

When something was delayed or brushed off, I leaned on skills I'd built in boardrooms and project war rooms:

- I asked specific questions:
    - "What is the next step?"
    - "Who owns this step?"
    - "When will it be done?"
- I showed up with data, not just feelings. Lab trends. Logs. Notes.
- And when necessary, I escalated, firmly but respectfully.

"This cannot wait. I need this addressed today."

Hospitals, insurance companies, and transplant centers are full of good people caught in bad systems. Their processes are fragile. Authorizations get lost. Orders expire. Messages sit in inboxes. The patients who do best are not the most compliant; they're the most engaged.

I treated the administrative side of my illness the way I'd manage a major enterprise project:

- **A master calendar** for labs, clearances, appointments, and refills.
- **A weekly review** to ask: What's pending? What's missing? What's about to expire?
- **PDF copies of everything**, labeled and backed up, not just "in the portal somewhere."

And I prepared for the call long before it came.

A go-bag sat ready with:
- Insurance cards and ID
- Medication list
- Comfortable clothes and toiletries
- Chargers
- A short list of who to notify

- Recent labs and key documents

Because when the phone rings and they say, "We have a kidney, can you be here in a few hours?", that is not the time to hunt for your wallet, your parking directions, or clean socks.

I learned to respect what each center did well:

- The **VA** moved slowly but cared deeply once you made it through the door.
- **Hartford Hospital** offered clarity, structure, and a transplant team that communicated like a well-drilled unit.
- **Yale** had brilliant surgeons and post-transplant expertise, but its size meant more bureaucracy and more follow-up from my side.

There is no perfect center. You survive by combining their strengths and filling in the gaps with your own discipline.

Staying Grounded When the Body Fails

The emotional skills that saved me weren't dramatic. No cinematic speeches. No triumphant soundtracks.

They were quiet: equanimity, acceptance, and emotional endurance.

Equanimity was learning to hold fear and hope in the same hand without letting either take over. Acceptance was not giving up; it was finally seeing reality clearly enough to make good decisions. And emotional endurance was the simple commitment to keep showing up, even when I had no idea what the next lab, call, or scan would bring.

On low-hope days, I didn't wait for inspiration. I leaned on routine:

- Make the bed. Order in the room created order in my head.
- Step outside, even briefly. Sunlight and air reminded me that the world continued beyond my body.
- Focus on the next milestone, not the entire road: "Make it to the next lab. The next visit. The next class."

Hope, I discovered, is less of an emotion and more of a discipline. Some days, I didn't feel hopeful at all. I just behaved as if hope still mattered, and eventually my emotions caught up.

Fear never fully leaves you. It just changes volume.

When labs dipped, or symptoms flared, fear tried to narrate the story: This is it. It's over. You're done. I learned to name it quickly:

"You're afraid because the numbers dropped. Fear is not fact."

Then I'd come back to what I could control: hydration, meds, rest, and calling the team. Fear thrives in ambiguity. It shrinks when you bring structure, truth, and action into the room.

Certain phrases and scriptures became anchors:
- "This too shall pass."
- "One day at a time."
- Psalm 46:10: "Be still, and know that I am God."
- And from the Navy: "Slow is smooth. Smooth is fast."

Courage, on most days, looked almost boring:
- Taking medications when I was sick of pills
- Drinking water when I didn't feel like it
- Showing up to appointments I wanted to cancel
- Teaching when fatigue felt like a second gravity

- Asking hard questions even when the answers scared me

That's the kind of courage that gets you to transplant, not big speeches, but small, consistent acts of faithfulness.

Journaling, simple prayers, and honest conversations with a few people who could hold the weight of my truth helped keep me aligned. They didn't erase the emotional pain, but they kept me from collapsing under it. They reminded me that I was still Daniel—not just a patient, not just an eGFR value on a chart.

Protecting the People You Love While You Fight Your War

Chronic illness does not happen to one person. It happens to a family.

The patient's suffering is visible: scars, labs, and IV lines. The spouse's suffering is quieter: watching, anticipating, absorbing, holding.

Spouses of chronically ill patients become everything at once:
- Emotional anchor
- Logistics coordinator
- Silent worrier
- Practical problem-solver

If I could speak to them directly, I'd say: You don't have to be superhuman. Be present. Your job is not to fix everything. Your job is to sit in the room and remind your partner they're still a person, not just a chart.

Marcia did that better than anyone.

She listened when there were no good answers. She showed up to appointments, to late-night worries, to hard conversations. She asked the doctors the questions I was too tired or too numb to articulate. At home, she protected peace. She didn't eliminate stress, but she refused to let sickness dominate the atmosphere.

Her presence was medicine.

We made mistakes, too. The biggest one couples make is trying to "protect" each other by hiding the truth. The sick partner hides symptoms to avoid worrying the family. The spouse hides fear to avoid adding weight. Silence grows. Distance follows.

Illness doesn't destroy relationships.
Silence does.

We learned to talk plainly, but calmly, to our kids:

"My numbers dropped a bit. Here's what that means. Here's what the doctors are doing. I'm still here. We're still a family. You are not responsible for fixing this."

Kids don't need medical granularity. They need emotional clarity and a sense of stability. They need to know there's a plan, that they are loved, and that their parent is still fighting.

The rituals mattered, maybe more than the big talks did:

- Family dinners, even if I was exhausted.
- Checking in about their days.
- Sunday rhythms.
- Movies on the couch.

These weren't attempts to pretend nothing was wrong. They were reminders that illness had entered our story, but it did not get to become the entire story.

On transplant day, all the emotions collided: fear, relief, gratitude, guilt, hope. There is no clean way to package that. The best preparation is honest expectation and open love:

- Expect emotional messiness.
- Talk through logistics: who goes to the hospital, who sends updates, who takes care of what at home.

- Say what you need to say before you're rolled down the hallway, not because you expect the worst, but because life-changing days deserve nothing unsaid.

A transplant is not just a surgery. It's a family event.

Work, Leadership, and Chronic Illness

For years, I lived a paradox: a chronically ill man functioning as if his body were fine.

Here's what I wish more professionals understood:
- You can be outstanding at your job and chronically ill at the same time.
- You cannot pretend your body is a non-factor.

I started treating my health priorities, hydration, labs, sleep, and meds, the same way I treated board meetings and strategy sessions: scheduled, protected, and non-negotiable. If you sacrifice them for work, eventually, work will be taken from you anyway, by force.

Instead of trying to maintain speed, I leaned into strategy:
- Prioritizing what only I could do
- Delegating aggressively
- Letting go of the myth that I had to be everywhere, for everyone, all the time

Disclosure at work became a matter of strategy, not confession. I told the people who needed to know:

- My immediate leader
- HR, for leave and accommodation purposes
- One or two trusted colleagues who could step in quickly

Everyone else? I kept it to myself, not out of shame, but out of wisdom. Not everyone can hold that information well. Not everyone should have it.

Healthy leadership while your body is under siege looks like:

- Calendar discipline, blocking out labs, rest, and medical calls
- Surgical prioritization, asking daily: What truly matters today?
- Clear communication, so your team isn't blindsided or confused.

Where I failed was where so many Type-A leaders fail: I treated symptoms as inconveniences, not warnings. I traveled too hard, worked through exhaustion, ignored rising blood pressure during high-stress weeks, and let "they need me" override "I need to live."

Those choices cost me kidney function.

Real resilience in leadership isn't about carrying everything on your back. It's about adapting your leadership so you don't break yourself or the people following you.

Chronically ill professionals bring something rare to the table: hard-won efficiency, perspective, and the ability to make clear decisions under pressure. They don't need pity. They need systems that make sustainable excellence possible.

Faith, Purpose, and Life After Transplant

The habits that held my soul together were not complicated. They were small and consistent:

- Short, honest prayers: "Give me strength for today."
- Stillness, even for a few minutes, before the noise of the day took over.
- Scripture in small doses, sometimes just a single line: "Be still, and know…"
- Gratitude, especially when I didn't feel like it: a good lab, a kind nurse, a stable BP reading, a quiet evening at home.

As my health declined, faith stopped being an idea and became a survival framework.

Prayer simplified. I stopped explaining the situation to God as if He needed my briefing. I stopped bargaining. Instead, it became: "Walk with me through this. Shape me in this. Don't let me waste whatever this is supposed to teach me."

Surrender shifted from philosophical to practical: I let go of outcomes I could not control and focused on the few I could. Purpose sharpened. When you're not sure how many years you have, your tolerance for nonsense drops quickly. Family, students, patients like you, the work that genuinely serves others, those things rise to the surface.

And then, after the transplant, everything shifted again.

Post-transplant life is blessed, but it is not casual.

The best practices are brutally straightforward:

- **Take every medication on time**. No exceptions. No "I forgot."
- **Hydrate as if the kidney depends on it—because it does**.
- **Protect yourself from infection**. Masks, handwashing, boundaries during flu season.
- **Sleep**. It's as medicinal as anything in the pill organizer.
- **Keep every appointment**. Labs reveal trouble long before symptoms do.

My new routines were simple:

- Walking daily, even when I felt "good enough" to sit.
- Tracking creatinine, tacrolimus levels, and trends so I knew my new baselines.

- Saying no to high-stress meetings, to unnecessary travel, to drama, to environments that could undo what surgery had just restored.

Boundaries were no longer negotiable. They were stewardship.

Stewardship, for me, means living in a way that honors the sacrifice behind this kidney. It means recognizing that Ryan's generosity is not just something I'm grateful for, it's something I'm accountable to.

Every pill I take on time, every glass of water, every follow-up I attend, every decision to rest instead of grind, every moment I choose peace over chaos, that's me honoring the man who gave up a piece of his body so I could stay in this world with my family.

Reflection — A Quiet Code for Moving Forward

If I had to boil everything in this chapter into a short "Resilience Code," it would sound something like this:

1. **Show up every day, especially when you don't want to.**
2. **Control what you can. Release what you can't.**
3. **Protect your health like your future depends on it, because it does.**
4. **Ask for help before you collapse.**
5. **Track the truth. Data beats denial.**

6. **Guard your mind from fear and cynicism.**

7. **Live as if someone else paid for your second chance, because in my case, someone did.**

For my children, for any reader walking a similar path, for the students who sit in my classroom and wonder how they'll navigate their own storms, I'd say this:

Life will break you at times. It broke me. It took my parents early. It took my brother. It almost took my kidneys. But it never took my purpose, because I refused to hand that over.

PKD changed my body. Transplant changed my life. Resilience changed how I live.

Surviving kept me breathing. Purpose made those breaths worth something.

If you take anything from my story, let it be this:

You may not get to choose your diagnosis, your setback, or your shadow. But you do get to choose your discipline. You do get to choose your habits. You do get to choose how you carry what you did not choose.

And sometimes, carrying it with faith, honesty, and love becomes the very light that outshines the shadow.

Chapter 12

Paying It Forward

The first time someone told me, "Your story helped me," I didn't quite know what to do with it.

For most of my life, I've been the one quietly pushing through: the sailor who followed orders, the technologist who solved problems, the professor who explained hard things in simple terms. I wasn't used to being the example. I certainly wasn't trying to be anyone's inspiration. I was trying to stay alive, love my family, do my work, and honor God with the time I had left.

But surviving what I survived, a nearly two-decade countdown from PKD to transplant, the surgery, the recovery, the "what ifs" and "not yets", did something inside of me. It shifted paying it forward from a nice idea to a non-negotiable responsibility.

I had been given more time. The question became: what would I do with it?

A Second Chance, A New Obligation

Before the transplant, "**service**" meant a lot of things to me: Navy duty, long hours at work, taking care of my family, and teaching my students. After the transplant, the word changed shape.

Service stopped being mostly about performance and started being about presence.

I realized I had walked through something that many people fear in the abstract and some face in the most concrete way imaginable: a failing body, an uncertain future, and the sense that your life might be tilting toward an early ending. I didn't read about it in a textbook; I lived it in hospital hallways, lab chairs, and quiet 3 a.m. worries.

When Ryan gave me his kidney, he didn't just keep me alive; he reset my compass. His choice, his gift, made it impossible to treat my survival as a private victory. It felt like God and another human being had conspired to hand me a second chance and then quietly asked, "Now what will you do with it?"

I couldn't answer that with titles or promotions. I had to answer it with how I showed up for other people.

First Ripples: My Daughter, My Colleagues, My Quiet Circle

The first person I really paid it forward to wasn't a stranger on the internet or a patient in a hospital waiting room. It was my own daughter.

Not long after my transplant, she received her own PKD diagnosis. I remember sitting with her in that exam room, watching the same kind of worry cross her face that I once saw in my own. The words I had heard years earlier, no cure, progressive, chronic— now echoed in a new generation.

In that moment, I wasn't soon to be Dr. O'Connell, or CIO, or professor. I was just a father with scars under his shirt who knew the terrain she was about to walk.

I didn't give her medical advice. That belongs to her doctors. What I gave her was something different:

I gave her presence.

I went with her to her appointments. I listened when she worried. I translated some of the language I had spent years learning, not to tell her what to do, but to make the road feel less foreign. I told her what I wish someone had told me early on:

You are allowed to be scared.
You are allowed to ask questions.
You are allowed to live a full life with this.

If my journey has any value, it's that she doesn't have to start from zero. She can look at my story and see that PKD is not the end of anything; it's the beginning of a different kind of strength.

Around the same time, old colleagues and friends began to reach out. Some were facing their own diagnoses, kidney-related or otherwise. Others were silently carrying medical fears that they had never spoken aloud. Somehow, hearing what I had walked through permitted them to open up.

We didn't sit down for formal counseling sessions. We talked on the phone. We texted. We met for coffee. I shared what it felt like to live in the in-between, between "you're sick" and "you're not done yet." I talked about lab days and waiting rooms, about how fear can make the hours longer and the nights louder.

I never said, "Do this."

More often, I said, "You're not crazy for feeling this way," and "You're not alone."

Sometimes the first step in healing is not a new medication or procedure. Sometimes it's simply being able to say, "I'm scared," and having someone answer, "Me too, and I'm still here."

The Classroom After Surgery

The classroom has always been one of my favorite places: whiteboard markers, questions, students half-worried about grades and half-worried about life.

After the transplant, the way I taught changed.

I still covered analytics, AI, data, and cybersecurity. I still cared about rigor and standards. But there was a new undercurrent to everything I did: an awareness that every person in that room was carrying something I couldn't see.

Having taught through fatigue, hidden pain, and fluctuating lab values, I began to look at my students differently. The young man staring blankly at his laptop might not be lazy; he might be exhausted from working two jobs. The student who missed class might not be indifferent; she might be caring for a sick parent, or fighting her own battle.

So I started weaving resilience into my lessons, not as a TED Talk, but as quiet truths:

- That resilience is rarely glamorous.
- That discipline shows up in the small decisions no one applauds.
- That success is not just about intellect, it's about endurance.

I didn't turn every lecture into a transplant story. But occasionally, when it fit, I'd mention that I'd been teaching in the shadow of a failing organ, or that I'd graded papers from a hospital bed. Not for sympathy, but to make something clear:

You can be going through something hard and still move forward. You can feel afraid and still show up.

When I finally told one of my classes that I'd be out for surgery, the room fell completely silent. Later, students emailed and said that watching me return, scarred, tired, but present, gave them a different picture of what strength looks like.

It isn't loud.
It isn't perfect.
It's consistent.

Leading With a Different Lens

In my professional life, I've always been wired for results: projects delivered, systems stable, teams aligned. The transplant didn't erase that drive, but it added a new lens.

I became more curious about what people were carrying beneath the surface.

When someone on my team seemed off, I no longer jumped straight to performance. I asked more questions. I made more space for real answers. I began gently insisting that people keep their medical appointments, go to the doctor, and take the day off if they needed it.

Health moved from a polite HR talking point to something I was willing to protect. I knew what it felt like to ignore symptoms for too long. I didn't want anyone on my watch to pay that price if it could be avoided.

My leadership shifted from "How do we hit this deadline?" to "How do we do this well and keep our people whole?"

I still expect excellence. But I no longer define excellence as squeezing the last ounce of energy out of someone. The transplant taught me the cost of that. It taught me that sometimes the bravest thing a person can do is admit, "I need help."

Now, when employees or colleagues go through illness, surgeries, or personal crises, I don't only ask, "Are you okay?" I ask, "What needs to change so you can carry this?" We adjust schedules, redistribute work, and extend grace.

It's not softness. It's stewardship.

Faith, Calling, and Quiet Courage

If you've read this far, you already know that faith has been the thread running under everything: diagnosis, decline, deployment, family, labs, and that long hallway toward the operating room.

The transplant didn't introduce God to my story. It revealed just how present He'd been all along.

I don't believe I was "lucky" to get a kidney on September 4, 2024, exactly seventeen years after my diagnosis. I believe that was grace within timing, only God fully understands.

Do I think God kept me alive for a reason? Yes.

Not because I'm special, but because He isn't finished with me yet.

That sense of calling doesn't show up as a voice from the clouds. It shows up in much quieter ways:

- A student who says, "Your story helped me book my own doctor's appointment."
- A veteran who admits he's been avoiding care and then decides to go.

- A fellow patient who texts late at night, terrified about their upcoming surgery.

In those moments, I remember the prayers whispered over hospital sheets, the verses taped to my bathroom mirror, the sense that I was being carried when I couldn't walk very far on my own.

Now, when I tell someone, "I'm praying for you," it's not a throwaway line. It's a memory of how prayer held me together when nothing else made sense.

I don't force faith on anyone. But I no longer hide that it's the backbone of my survival.

What I Share With Patients and Families

Because of what I've been through, people sometimes ask me questions about kidneys, lab results, transplants, or PKD. I always start with a simple truth:

I'm not your doctor. I can't give medical advice.

What I can share is what helped me navigate my own road—not as instructions, but as perspective.

I tell people that advocating for themselves is not rude or disrespectful; it's necessary. Ask questions until you understand. Bring someone with you to appointments if the information feels overwhelming. Write things down. Speak up if something doesn't sit right.

I encourage them to learn enough about their condition to spot patterns: how their body responds, what their labs tend to do, what "normal" feels like for them. Not so they can replace their doctors, but so they can partner with them.

When families ask what to do, I don't hand them a checklist. I tell them what mattered most to me:

The people who didn't disappear when things got complicated. The ones who sat and listened without trying to fix everything. The ones who stayed consistent when the process was long and the outcome uncertain.

The worst part of chronic illness isn't always pain; it's feeling like you are carrying it alone.

If my story gives anyone a blueprint, I hope it's for this: how to show up. How to stand beside someone in the valley without pretending the valley isn't real.

Honoring Ryan, Honoring the Gift

I think about Ryan's kidney every day, not in a fearful way, but in a grateful one. It hums quietly in my body, doing work my original organs could no longer do.

When he once said, "You do so much for others," it struck me deeply. Because in my mind, I was just doing what I could to stay afloat and help where I was able. His words reframed that. They felt less like a compliment and more like a charge:

Keep going.

I honor his gift in very practical ways: I take my medications. I show up to follow-up appointments. I pay attention to my body. I try to manage stress instead of ignoring it. I respect the limits that weren't there when I was twenty-five.

But I also honor his gift in less visible ways.

Every time I step into a classroom, sit with a student in office hours, listen to a colleague who's overwhelmed, or talk with someone who's newly diagnosed, I bring his generosity with me. His decision didn't just extend my life; it multiplied my capacity to serve.

I can't ever pay him back, not really. What I can do is live in a way that makes his sacrifice worth it.

Legacy, Lighthouses, and the Long View

Transplant forces you to think about legacy, whether you want to or not.

When my kids look back on this season, I don't want them to remember a man who was defined by sickness. I want them to remember a father who kept showing up, even when he was tired or afraid. A man who didn't pretend to be invincible, but who refused to quit.

I hope my daughter, as she walks her own PKD journey, sees more than lab reports and medical terms. I hope she sees a living example that a diagnosis is not a finish line; it's a call to live differently, more deliberately, more aware of what matters.

For strangers who may read this one day, patients, caregivers, students, veterans, anyone standing at the edge of their own quiet war, I don't need to be remembered by name. If my story serves as a lighthouse when the water gets rough, that's enough.

I want this memoir to whisper something simple but stubborn into their darkness:

"If he could survive this, maybe I can survive mine."

If I Could Give You One Thing

If I could hand you one thing from my journey, it wouldn't be a strategy or a slogan. It would be this conviction:

You are stronger than you think.

Not because strength erases fear or pain, but because it often grows in the exact moments you're sure you have nothing left.

I would hand you the belief that your story isn't over, not even if the news is bad, the path is hard, and the road ahead is unclear.

I would hand you the certainty that you don't have to walk it alone.

There is help. There is community. There is faith. There is a way forward, even when you can't see all of it yet.

My own quiet war has taken me through disease, grief, guilt, falls, surgery, and recovery. It has also taken me through love, redemption, service, teaching, friendship, and grace.

If anything in these pages stays with you, let it be this:

Hope is not naïve. It's necessary. Grit is not about never breaking; it's about getting back up. Faith does not guarantee an easy road; it guarantees you won't walk it alone.

And paying it forward?

That's how we honor the time we're given, by turning our survival into someone else's courage.

Reflection – Living the Gift Forward

When I look back at everything that led to this chapter, the diagnosis, the slow decline, the transplant, the recovery, the conversations in quiet corners and hospital hallways, I see a pattern I couldn't see at the time.

None of it was wasted.

The pain was real. The fear was real. The uncertainty was real. But so were the people who showed up, the prayers whispered, the small mercies in ordinary days. Somewhere along the way, survival stopped being just about staying alive and became about learning how to live *for* something and *for* someone beyond myself.

Paying it forward is not a grand gesture. It's not a slogan or a campaign. It is the daily decision to let what you've been through soften you instead of harden you, to let it open your heart instead of closing it. It is choosing presence over performance, listening over fixing, service over self-protection.

I don't share my story because I see myself as a hero. I share it because I know what it's like to be on the other side of the table, staring at lab results you don't fully understand, wondering if your body is going to hold out, trying to look brave for the people who love you. I remember the loneliness of it. I also remember the people who refused to let me carry it alone.

In my second life, legacy isn't a monument or a résumé line. Legacy is a ripple. It's my daughter knowing she is not walking her PKD journey in the dark. It's a student deciding to make that doctor's appointment finally. It's a veteran choosing to ask for help. It's a colleague exhaling when they realize they don't have to be indestructible to be valued.

If you carry anything from this chapter into your own life, I hope it's this: you don't have to wait for a perfect moment, an ideal plan, or a perfect version of yourself to start paying it forward. You can begin with what you have, where you are, with the story you already carry.

Your scars do not disqualify you from helping others; they qualify you to walk beside them.

Some days, paying it forward will look like a big decision. Most days, it will look like something small: a phone call returned, a text answered, a chair pulled up next to someone who is quietly breaking. Those things may not look dramatic from the outside, but I can tell you, from the perspective of someone who has been on the receiving end, they can be the difference between despair and hope.

I was given more time. I intend to spend it making sure that someone else feels less alone in their own quiet war.

That, to me, is what paying it forward really is: turning the miracle of still being here into a reason someone else decides to keep going.

VI

The Meaning

Chapter 13

After the Second Life

The first moments after a transplant don't feel cinematic. They feel strange, disorienting, and holy in ways you don't fully understand at the time. When consciousness returned, it wasn't gradual; it hit in fragments.

Light.
Blinding at first.
A sharp white glare pushes through my eyelids.

Then blur.
Shapes without edges, outlines without meaning.

And then, almost suddenly, the room dimmed. Not darkness, just softer. Calmer. As if the world had turned down its volume so my spirit could ease back into the body that had just been opened, repaired, and rewired for a second chance at life.

I remember blinking hard, trying to anchor myself. I remember the pressure in my abdomen reminding me that something inside me was new, foreign, yet already working.

And my first actual thought wasn't about me.

I hope Ryan is okay.

It was an instinctive reflex, concern for the man who had just gone through surgery on my behalf. Before I wondered about the kidney, the labs, or even my own survival, my heart went out to him. Was he awake? Was he comfortable? Did he make it through without complications?

That moment revealed something I didn't expect:
This second life wasn't mine alone.
It belonged to two families. Two stories. Two journeys are now permanently connected.

Understanding What Happened Inside Me

Once the haze lifted, curiosity took over. I've always been someone who tries to understand the mechanics of what's happening around me, and inside me.

For nearly two decades, PKD had slowly undermined my kidneys. Cysts grew, silently and relentlessly, turning once-smooth organs into clusters of fluid-filled chambers. They didn't fail suddenly; they declined like an hourglass running out of sand.

Here's what I came to understand about the transplant, not as medical advice, but as meaning:

1. **My native kidneys stayed inside me.** They weren't removed because taking them out would have caused more trauma, more blood loss, more risk. They would remain where they were, scarred, enlarged, and silent witnesses to the years I fought to stay ahead of CKD.

2. **The new kidney was placed in my lower abdomen.** I learned that transplanted kidneys usually go in the front, tucked near the pelvis, connected to fresh vessels and plumbing. It still amazes me that the body can accept a kidney in an entirely new location and immediately start working with it.

3. **The renal artery and vein were connected with careful precision.** The blood flow was the key. Once circulation reached the kidney, it woke up. In many cases, transplanted kidneys produce urine right on the operating table. Mine did. I didn't know it then, but later, hearing it described felt like hearing the sound of life returning.

4. **The ureter was joined to my bladder like a new chapter being stitched into an old book.** Not perfect, not original, but functional, living, and full of possibility.

5. **Immunosuppression became part of my daily covenant.** The body is loyal, sometimes too loyal. It wants to reject anything unfamiliar. These medications teach it to accept miracles as usual.

Each pill, each dosage, each schedule is not just a treatment; it's a partnership between discipline and grace.

The First Nights: A Quiet Battle

The first night in recovery felt both peaceful and intense. Machines beeped steadily. Doctors and nurses came and went with purposeful calm. Every few hours, they checked vitals, labs, and output.

I wasn't scared.
I wasn't overwhelmed.
I was present.

For the first time in a long time, I wasn't fighting decline; I was fighting to rise. I was experiencing a rebound.

The difference is profound.

Pain came in waves, but it wasn't the pain of sickness; it was the pain of rebuilding. Not pain in the acute sense, but more of being swollen. Incisions throbbed. Muscles protested. The new kidney felt heavy at first, like a guest who needed time to settle in.

But the labs, those numbers I had spent years tracking, began moving in the opposite direction for the first time in seventeen years.

Creatinine dropping.

BUN stabilizing.

eGFR rising.

It was as if someone had turned back the internal clock.

The Quiet Gratitude of a Family Man

My kids are grown, but that doesn't lessen the bond. It deepens it. They worry differently. They love differently. They watch closely.

As I recovered, I wasn't fighting for the chance to raise young children; I was fighting to *continue being part of their adult lives:*

their milestones

their futures

their careers

their families someday

the simple privilege of watching them grow into the people they're becoming

The transplant didn't restart my life; it renewed my role.

When I saw my family walk into the room, cautious, hopeful, relieved, the meaning of survival shifted. This wasn't just my story. It was ours. It was about continuity. About remaining present. About stewarding the time I'd been given to keep showing up, guiding, supporting, loving, and living alongside the people who matter most.

I wasn't trying to be a hero.
I wasn't trying to be inspirational.
I was simply trying to be here.
A father.
A husband.
A son.
A brother.
A man who still had work to do.

A Donor's Gift and the Weight of Honor

The first time I saw Ryan after the surgery, he was sitting up, smiling, recovering at his own pace. Relief washed through me. Gratitude that exceeded words.

People talk about "heroism," but Ryan never saw it that way. He saw it as an act of faith, friendship, and humanity. And I saw it as a responsibility.

His gift didn't just extend my life—it deepened its meaning.

I didn't feel guilty.
I felt stewardship.

A need to:

- walk wisely

- live gratefully

- serve generously

- honor the sacrifice

- and respect the body I now carry

Every time I hydrate, rest, or take medication, I'm honoring him. Every time I teach, mentor, or support someone, I'm living the purpose he helped me continue.

His kidney keeps me alive.
His generosity keeps me accountable.

Understanding Matching Without Making It Clinical

I learned enough to appreciate the complexity without pretending to be a doctor.

Matches aren't about perfection, they're about compatibility:

- blood type

- HLA markers

- Antibodies

- crossmatching

What amazed me wasn't the science itself, but the orchestration behind it. That two people, with different backgrounds, different bloodlines, could align in a way that allows one life to strengthen another.

It made me see God's hand not as distant but deeply involved.
Not abstract but orchestrated.
Not random but intentional.

How Immunosuppression Became a Spiritual Practice

I never imagined taking medication could feel sacred. Yet each morning and evening, as I lined up my pills, I felt the weight of stewardship.

These medications weren't burdens.
They were bridges, connecting my body to the gift it received.

They prevented rejection.
They protected life.

They symbolized the partnership between me, the donor, the medical team, and God's provision.

Some days I felt strong.
Some days, my body felt the side effects.

But every day, the routine reminded me of grace stitched into science.

Stepping Back into the World

When I returned to work and teaching, I did so slowly—but with clarity. The world looked different:

Colors sharper.
Conversations deeper.
Time heavier.
Purpose clearer.

My transplant didn't turn me into a different person. It refined the person I already was.

I became more patient.
More intentional.
More grateful.
More steady.
More present.

I didn't rush anymore. I didn't take days for granted. I didn't push past limits in the ways I once did. Healing teaches a man that strength isn't proven through exhaustion, it's proven through wisdom.

The Gift of the Second Life: Not Bigger, But Deeper

I expected a second life to feel... grand. Cinematic. Dramatic.

But it wasn't.

It was quieter.
Simpler.
More grounded.
More human.

A second life doesn't ask you to reinvent yourself.
It asks you to live with clearer eyes and a steadier heart.

It asks you to:

- value what matters
- release what doesn't
- give more freely
- love more openly
- forgive more quickly
- and live more intentionally

I don't measure my second life in milestones.
I measure it in moments.

Walking without fatigue.

Teaching without exhaustion.

Praying with focus.

Breathing with gratitude.

Seeing my family with a fresh perspective.

This life feels less like a continuation and more like a calibration, an alignment of purpose.

Reflection — The Sacred Ordinary of a Borrowed Life

When I think of this chapter, this second life, I don't see the surgery table or the machines or the monitors. I see the quiet moments:

- the dimming lights as I woke up
- the first deep breath that didn't feel heavy
- the relief when I knew Ryan was okay
- the steady hands of nurses who did their work with quiet excellence
- the whispered prayers in the dark
- the first lab values are moving in the right direction
- the grateful weight of knowing God extended my time

This second life is not loud.

It is not dramatic.

It is not flashy.

It is sacred.

It is ordinary in the most extraordinary way.

It is hours and days and sunrises I wasn't guaranteed, but was given.
Time I intend to honor.
Time I intend to use well.
Time I carry with reverence.

I woke up after my transplant in a blur of light and confusion. But today, I see everything clearly:

- This second life is not owed.

- It is not accidental.

- It is not random.

-

It is grace, stitched through science, anchored by faith, and carried forward with gratitude.

And I intend to live every borrowed sunrise with purpose.

Chapter 14

The Things I Wish I Knew

When I look back at the earliest days of my diagnosis, those first confusing, disorienting moments in 2007, I sometimes wish I could sit beside the man I was back then. Not to warn him, not to frighten him, but to whisper something that would have loosened the knot in his chest, softened the fear in his wife's eyes, and steadied the ground under his feet.

I wish I could have said: **"Have faith. This will work out. Not easily, not quickly, but faithfully."**

That simple truth would have changed so much. It wouldn't have removed the disease or erased the uncertainty. Still, it would have given us something we desperately needed: hope that had structure, shape, and direction.

In the beginning, I thought chronic illness meant immediate decline. That everything would stop at once. That life would become a series of hospital visits until the inevitable ending arrived sooner than expected. I thought PKD would collapse everything: my career, my identity, my ability to provide, my future with my family.

But that was a misconception, not the truth.

Chronic illness does not announce itself with a finish line. It introduces itself as a question you must learn to live inside. What I wish I knew then is that PKD was not the end of my story. It was the beginning of a different kind of strength, one that was slow, deliberate, intimate, and profoundly human.

What Fear Looks Like the First Time

Fear arrives in strange ways. Sometimes it's loud. Sometimes it's silent. But it always finds its way in.

For me, fear first visited as the unknown.

Not just fear for myself, fear for my family.

Would I be able to walk my daughter down the aisle? Would I be there for my sons? Would I be able to keep working, keep teaching, keep leading? Would my wife have to carry more than she ever deserved?

I thought fear would make me crumble.
Instead, it made me sharper.

Even in denial, even in the early shock, something inside me began to calibrate. Not overnight, but gradually. I shifted from panic to process, from chaos to clarity. I became calm, collected, and deliberate because I had to be. Because survival wasn't just biology, it was discipline, faith, structure, and choosing forward motion on days when everything felt frozen.

I didn't know that the emotional landscape would be as challenging as the physical one. What surprised me most wasn't the fear itself. It was realizing how invisible illness can distort identity, dignity, and morale.

People who love you don't always understand what they can't see.

Colleagues don't always recognize the battle behind the smile.

Friends don't always know how to engage with something they can't fix.

I wish I had known earlier how heavy that emotional load can become.

And I wish I had shown myself more grace.

The Cost of Pushing Too Hard

As a Navy veteran, a technologist, an executive, and someone who has always worked without excuses, I believed fatigue was something you outworked, not something you honored.

I believed rest was optional.

I pushed myself through exhaustion that should have stopped me in my tracks. I went to work when I should have stayed home. I taught when my energy was drained. I traveled when my body was signaling loudly for me to slow down. I kept too much inside because

I didn't want to burden anyone.

What I wish I knew then is simple:
Rest is not surrender. Rest is a strategy.
Fatigue is not weakness. Fatigue is a warning.
And ignoring the warnings does not make you stronger; it makes you vulnerable.

Recovering from my transplant showed me how far I had pushed my body beyond its limits. The surge of clarity and energy afterward was both exhilarating and humbling. It made me realize just how fragile I had become and how much I had normalized exhaustion.

Had I known then what I know now, I would have honored rest the way I honored discipline: as a critical part of survival.

The Spiritual Cost and Strength of the Journey

Chronic illness doesn't only reshape your schedule; it reshapes your spirit.

I wish I had understood earlier that faith is not just belief; it is endurance. It is the ability to trust that you are being guided even when the map looks blank. It is learning that prayer is not a request; it is a relationship. It is remembering that God is present even when the outcome is unclear.

What I know now is this:
Illness can strip away your physical strength, but it also exposes your inner one.
It can make you feel isolated, but it can deepen your connection to God.
It can frighten you, but it can refine you.

In the quiet hours, late nights, early mornings, waiting rooms, and lab chairs, I learned that faith is not decorative. It is functional. It is oxygen.

I wish I knew back then that spiritual resilience would become the backbone of my journey.

The Importance of Fighting for Yourself

I didn't know, at first, how crucial it was to advocate for myself.

To ask questions.

To understand the numbers.

To speak up even when I felt intimidated.

To say, "Explain that again."

No one told me that clarity wasn't automatic—that you have to fight for it.

What I wish I knew is this:
Doctors are experts, but they don't live inside your body.
You are the steward of your health.

You must be your own advocate, your own historian, your own voice.

Advocating for yourself isn't confrontation.

It is survival with dignity.

I wish I had embraced that sooner.

What Illness Does to a Family

I wish I knew how much this journey would affect the people I love.

The emotional strain on my wife.

The uncertainty on my children's faces.

The silent weight carried by everyone around me.

Chronic illness enters every room before you do.
It affects marriages, family rhythms, finances, responsibilities, moods, and hope.

It isn't that families don't want to help.

It's that they often don't know how.

I wish I had known earlier to communicate more. To tell them when I was scared instead of pretending to be invincible. To share what I was feeling rather than letting them guess. To let them into the process rather than carrying it alone.

I also wish I knew how deeply my illness would shape my children, not just emotionally, but practically and spiritually.

Even more, I wish I had known that one day, my daughter would sit in a medical exam room hearing the same diagnosis I heard years before… and that my presence would be part of her courage.

Being Too Hard on Myself

There were countless moments when I was my own harshest critic.

Sitting in my truck between appointments.

Walking into my office, I was exhausted.

Staring at lab results that felt like report cards from an unrelenting universe.

I kept telling myself what I should be doing, what I could be doing, why I wasn't doing more. I forgot that survival itself was labor. I forgot that the body has limits. I forgot that being human is not a flaw.

Looking back, I wish I had been more patient with myself.
More forgiving.
More understanding.
More human.

What I Wish Leaders Knew About Invisible Illness

If I could gather every leader, every boss, every executive I encountered along the way, I'd tell them this:
Invisible illness is real.
And the people you depend on might be fighting battles you cannot see.

Many leaders care about results more than people.

But good leaders understand that people make results possible.

I wish leaders knew:
You cannot push someone past their limits and expect excellence. You cannot ignore the human condition and expect

loyalty. You cannot treat employees like machines and expect them to stay.

Jobs come and go.

Organizations rise and fall.

But the people who give their time and strength are irreplaceable. Invisible illness is not laziness. It is not a lack of commitment. It is not a personal flaw. It is a fight. Often a quiet one.

I hope this chapter helps someone in leadership see the difference.

What Caregivers Never Hear Enough

To the caregivers, the wives, husbands, children, parents, friends, I wish I knew how to say, early on:
You matter more than you realize.

Caregivers don't simply help; they absorb. They stretch themselves. They sacrifice sleep, time, energy, and emotional stability. They are the anchor when the patient is drifting.

I wish I knew earlier how to express gratitude, not just for the big things, but for the thousand quiet acts that made my survival possible.

I wish caregivers knew this journey takes a toll on them, too. Their exhaustion is real. Their frustration is normal. Their emotional fatigue is not failure.

Caregivers deserve compassion, understanding, and support just as much as the patient.

The Truth That Hit Me Hardest After Transplant

After my transplant, when the fog cleared and the energy returned, I realized a truth that struck deeper than anything I'd felt before:
I had been far closer to death than I ever admitted.

The difference between the body I had before surgery and the body I had after was unmistakable. It wasn't subtle. It was dimensional, like moving from black-and-white to color, from static to clarity, from survival to life.

I suddenly felt thirty years younger. Focused. Renewed. Alive.

Another truth surprised me: healing takes time. More time than I wanted. More patience than I had. "Slow is smooth, and smooth is fast." I learned that the body has its own schedule. And rushing it only leads backward.

To The Newly Diagnosed: What I Wish I Could Tell You

If I could speak to someone who just heard the words "You have PKD," I'd say it with all sincerity:

Hold on.

It will be okay.

Not easy.

Not painless.

But okay.

PKD is a slow mover.

You will have time.

You will adapt.

You will learn.

You will live.

This diagnosis is overwhelming. It feels like a tidal wave. But hidden inside the fear is a road, long, winding, and real. You are not alone. You are not broken. And you are not without hope. Take me as proof.

Seventeen years passed between my diagnosis and transplant. Seventeen years of work, teaching, leadership, family, faith, and survival.

Your story is not over.

Not today.

Not with this diagnosis.

You have more chapters ahead.

Reflection – The Truth That Arrives Late

If I could gather every lesson from these years, the fear, the fatigue, the grace, the faith, the discipline, the family moments, the late-night doubts, the small victories, and distill them into something you could carry in your hands, I would offer you this:

You don't have to know everything today.
You only need to keep going.

The things I wish I knew back then were not secrets someone kept from me; they were truths that could only reveal themselves through lived experience. Through walking the long road. Through being humbled, strengthened, stretched, and renewed.

Chronic illness does not end your life. It recalibrates it. It reshapes your priorities. It redefines your strength. It teaches you who you are in the moments that demand everything.

If this chapter leaves any imprint on your heart, let it be this:
You are stronger than your fear.
You are more capable than your doubt.
You are more resilient than your circumstances.
And you do not walk alone.

The things I wish I knew have become the things I now offer forward, not as instruction, not as advice, but as testimony. A reminder that even in the hardest chapters, there is still purpose. Still direction. Still grace. Still a reason to believe that life is not finished with you yet. And if you ever feel unsteady, overwhelmed, or lost, remember:

Hope is still here.

Faith is still here.

Courage is still here.

So are you.

Chapter 15

Letters

There are things we live through that cannot be explained in conversation. Some truths only reveal themselves when put into words, quietly, intentionally, without interruption. As I reached this point in my story, I realized there were messages I had carried inside me for years. Gratitude I never fully expressed. Lessons I wanted to hand forward. Love, I wanted to name out loud.

This chapter is my way of doing that.

These letters are not polished speeches. They are not metaphors or crafted scenes. They are honest moments, written to the people who shaped my life, stood beside me, carried me, believed in me, or waited for me to come back.

Some of these letters can never be delivered.

But they still needed to be written.

Letter to Ryan

Dear Ryan,

There are not enough pages in this book to hold what I feel when I think of what you did for me. A kidney is not a gift someone gives lightly. It is not a shirt, not a tool, not a favor. It is a piece of yourself, your literal life, that you entrusted to me.

When I woke up after surgery, blurry-eyed under the bright lights, feeling the world come back into focus, my first thought was simple:

I hope he's okay.

I hoped your surgery went smoothly, that your pain was minimal, that your spirit was steady.

Your choice restored years to my life, years I can spend loving my family, working, teaching, serving, and simply waking up without the weight and fog of a failing organ. You gave me margin. Strength. Time. You gave me the chance to be here.

But more than that, you changed how I live. I carry your generosity with me every single day, quietly, humbly, gratefully. I honor your sacrifice when I take my medication, when I go to my appointments, when I make decisions that protect the life you helped extend.

You once said I "do so much for others," but truthfully, your act has enabled me to do even more.

Thank you, my friend.

For your courage.

Your compassion.

Your sacrifice.

Your belief that my life was worth extending.

I will spend the rest of my days living in a way that honors what you gave.

With gratitude beyond words,
Dan

Letter to My Wife

My love,

There are parts of this journey that only you witnessed. The middle-of-the-night fears. The exhaustion in my voice on days when I tried to hide it. The quiet moments where I wondered how much longer my body could carry me. You held more than I ever said out loud.

You were the calm in the chaos. The steadiness when everything else felt uncertain.

The voice that kept saying, "We'll get through this," even when the path looked impossible.

I wish I could go back and ease some of the burden you carried alone. So much of the emotional labor fell on you: worry, planning, managing, hoping, praying. You were my anchor long before the transplant, and you remained my anchor after.

When I think of survival, I don't think of numbers or lab values. I think of you.

Your patience. Your belief in me. Your willingness to love me through a season neither of us asked for.

Thank you for standing beside me, not just in the hospital, but in the everyday moments that felt just as heavy. Thank you for loving me when I felt fragile. Thank you for reminding me that illness does not erase identity, or worth, or joy.

You helped save my life, too, in ways no surgeon ever could.
Love Always,
Dan

Letter to All My Kids

To my children,

You may not fully realize how much your presence kept me going. I thought about you during every lab, every appointment, every sleepless night. I thought about your futures, your dreams, and your own families someday. I wanted to be there, to watch you grow, to guide you, to celebrate the milestones we take for granted until they are threatened.

When I felt tired, you gave me purpose.
When I felt discouraged, you gave me reason.
When I felt afraid, you reminded me why I needed to keep moving.

I want you to know something that took me years to learn:
Strength is not the absence of fear. Strength is choosing to move forward anyway.

I carried you in my heart through all of this, and I carry you still. You were never the weight. You were the reason.

With all my love,
Dad

Letter to My Daughter, Marissa

Dear Marissa,

Watching you receive the same diagnosis I heard years ago was one of the most challenging moments of my life. I would've absorbed it for you if I could. I would've shielded you. I would've stood between you and every ounce of fear.

But what struck me in that exam room wasn't your worry; it was your strength. Strength that reminded me of what I had to learn the hard way.

I want you to know this:

PKD does not define you. It does not limit your future. It does not shrink your worth.

You are powerful. You are capable. You are resilient in ways you may not fully see yet. You carry my story, but you are writing your own, and yours will be filled with victories I never imagined.

I will walk this road with you step by step. You will never face this alone.

I love you more than I can ever express.

Dad

Letter to My Son, Kevin

Dear Kevin,

You've always had a quiet steadiness about you, a strength that isn't loud, but deep. Through my journey, you watched, listened, and supported in your own thoughtful ways. You may not know how much that meant.

When things were difficult, just knowing you were in my corner made the load lighter.

I want you to remember this as you move through life: **It is okay to ask for help. It is OK to rest. It is OK to be human.**

Your gentleness is not weakness. Your empathy is not frailty. Those traits are gifts, not just to others, but to yourself.

I am proud of you.

Always.

Love,
Dad

Letter to My Son, Zachary

Zachary,

There is an energy in you, a spark, that has always reminded me of my younger self. Even when I was sick, your enthusiasm pulled me forward. You helped me stay engaged with the world when fatigue tried to drag me inward.

You gave me laughter during moments that felt too heavy. You gave me a distraction when I needed it most. You gave me joy in the middle of uncertainty.

I want you to carry this truth with you:
Life is unpredictable, but joy is worth fighting for.

Protect that spark. Nurture it. Let it guide you, not just in good seasons, but in the difficult ones too.

I am grateful God made me your father.

Love,
Dad

Letter to My Younger Self

To the man sitting in the doctor's office in 2007,

I know what you're thinking:
"This can't be happening."
"This will ruin everything."
"What will this mean for my family?"

You feel fear. You feel denial. You feel the weight of a future suddenly rewritten.

So let me tell you something you can't believe yet:
You will make it.
You will survive this season and the ones after it.
You will become stronger than the fear that grips you today.

One day, you'll look back and realize you didn't just endure, you grew, you served, you led, you loved, you lived. Have faith. Have patience. Give yourself grace.

God will carry you further than you think.

With compassion,
Your future self

Letter to My Older Self

To the man I hope to become,

I pray you are still walking with gratitude. I hope you continue to remember the gift you received, the time, the second chance, the clarity.

I hope you still honor Ryan's sacrifice with every choice you make.

I hope you still take your health seriously, not with fear, but with discipline.

I hope you are still present with your family, still teaching, still mentoring, still serving.

And I hope you never stop paying it forward.

If you've slowed down, rest. If you've lost perspective, return to gratitude. If you've forgotten the fragility of life, place your hand over your scar and remember the miracle.

Live well, old man.
You've earned it.

With hope,

Your younger, grateful self

Letter to My Parents

Dear Mom and Dad,

I find myself writing this letter long after both of you have left this world, but I feel you here in ways I never could have appreciated when I was younger. Time has a way of softening sharp edges, clarifying what mattered, and revealing the sacrifices that were invisible to a child and only fully understood by a grown man looking back.

You didn't have easy lives. You didn't come from wealth, privilege, or comfort. You taught me the kind of resilience that is earned, not inherited. You gave me discipline, a work ethic, and a belief that no circumstance was too heavy to lift with enough faith and determination. Those lessons carried me through deployments, medical verdicts, scans, fear, and a transplant that came seventeen years after the day the doctor first said "PKD."

Mom, I remember your softness, even in the moments you thought you weren't soft at all. You worried over us the way only a mother does, quietly, constantly, and thoroughly. I didn't always understand the depth of that love until I became a father. Now I see it in every moment I fear for my own children, in every silent prayer I send upward, in every long night spent wondering how to protect the people I love.

Dad, you were a man of steadiness, sometimes too stoic, sometimes too proud, but always present in your way. You taught me loyalty, commitment, and showing up even when life feels heavy. If I didn't say it enough when you were here, I know now just how much you carried so that we could feel safe. That kind of strength doesn't disappear; I take it with me still.

I wish you had been here to see the years that followed, your grandchildren being born, the children growing, my career unfolding, my journey through illness and transplant. I wish I could have told you about the fear and the fight, about the grace that kept me going, about Ryan's gift and the way it reset the trajectory of my life. But I also believe you've seen all of it from a place where nothing goes unnoticed and nothing is wasted.

If there is anything I wish I could give you now, it is this: the acknowledgment that your sacrifices were not in vain. I am who I am because of what you built in me. And I hope that in the way I live, serve, lead, and love, I honor you both, not perfectly, but truthfully.

Thank you for everything you poured into me, what you taught me, even the pieces I didn't understand until much later. Thank you for making me. Thank you for being there while you were around.

Will always miss you. Never forgotten. Your legacy and memory carry on.

Your son,
Dan

Letter to My Brother Jim

Dear Jim,

There is no easy way to write this letter, because our story was never simple. We weren't the kind of brothers who always saw eye to eye, and we both carried stubbornness that sometimes kept us apart longer than it should have. Our relationship had cracks, some small, some deep, and for years, we walked parallel lives that rarely touched.

But when your cancer came calling, all of that faded into the background. The distance, the disagreements, the stubborn silences, they suddenly felt small compared to the battle you were fighting. What mattered was that you were my brother, and you were suffering, and I needed to be there.

Standing by your bedside in those last days, I saw you differently. Not through the lens of old arguments or gaps we never filled, but as a man fighting with everything he had left. You faced breast cancer with a quietness that I'm still trying to understand. Even when your body weakened, there was something unbroken in you, something determined, something brave.

I've thought many times about what I should have said.

What we never talked about.

What I wish we had known how to say sooner.

But in those final days, the need for explanations disappeared. What remained was family, and love, and the simple truth that no matter how complicated our history was, the bond never broke completely.

Losing you forced me to see my own reflection more honestly. It made me confront the fragility of time, how quickly everything can change, how sickness makes all our old walls seem pointless. Your battle with cancer sharpened my awareness of my own illness, my own fears, my own race against the clock.

If I could talk to you now, I'd tell you this:

I'm sorry for the times we let pride win.

I'm grateful for the moments we did share.

And I'm honored I could stand with you at the end.

I hope you found peace in those final moments, the kind no one can take away. And I hope you know that, despite everything, the distance, the disagreements, the imperfections, I loved you. I still do.

I carry your memory with me, not as a wound, but as a reminder: Life is too short to hold onto old divides,

Faith is stronger than pride, and family is still family, even when it's complicated.

Rest now, Jim.
Your fight is over.
I'll keep going, with gratitude for the time we had, even the imperfect parts.

Your brother,
Daniel

Letter to My Transplant Team

To the entire team who cared for me,

There are no words that fully capture my gratitude. You weren't just professionals doing a job; you were the hands and minds God used to preserve my life.

Thank you for your skill. Your vigilance. Your compassion. Your precision. Your willingness to shoulder the responsibility of another human being's future.

You saw me not as a case, but as a person, with a family, a career, a life still unfolding. Your work restored more than organ function. It restored possibility.

Please know this:
Your work echoes far beyond hospital walls.

Every day of my second life carries your fingerprints.

With deep respect and gratitude,
Daniel O'Connell

Letter to Future Transplant Patients

To you, who stands where I once stood,

I won't pretend the road is easy. It isn't. It is long, uncertain, emotional, and at times overwhelming.

But I want to tell you something true:
You can do this.
You are stronger than you know.
And there is hope on the other side.

You will fear the surgery. You will worry about the future. You will wonder if your life will ever feel normal again. It will. Not instantly. Not perfectly. But beautifully.

There will be a day when you wake up and realize:
"I feel alive again."

The fog will lift. Your energy will return. Your purpose will sharpen. Do not walk this journey alone.

Reach out.

Ask for help.

Let people in.

And when you make it through, and you will, remember to support the next person standing where you stand now. You are not alone. You are not broken. You are becoming.

With courage and compassion,
Daniel

Reflection – What These Letters Really Mean

Writing these letters reminded me of something I didn't fully understand until now:

People shaped every chapter of my life.

By the ones who stood beside me.

By the ones who taught me.

By the ones who challenged me.

By the ones who saved me.

None of us survives alone.

None of us heals alone.

None of us rises alone.

These letters are my thank you, my apology, my encouragement, my confession, and my hope, bound together in the only way that felt honest.

If you take anything from this chapter, let it be this:

Love is not something we feel quietly.

It is something we speak, name, honor, and give.

Especially while we still can.

And if writing these letters taught me one final truth, it is this:

A life survives on medicine, but people restore it.

Chapter 16

After the War

There is a moment after any long battle, military, medical, or emotional, when everything becomes quiet. Not peaceful, not yet. Just quiet. A kind of stillness you don't fully trust at first, because you've grown accustomed to alarms, to waiting for the next hit of bad news, to living in a state of readiness that never quite lets you exhale.

But eventually, slowly, something shifts.

The war stops demanding your attention.
Your body stops sending distress signals.
Your days stop revolving around numbers, appointments, and what-ifs.

And you begin to realize you've entered a chapter you never thought you'd reach:

Life after survival.

For years, I had been preparing for crisis, for decline, for transplant. I was prepared for procedures, for pain, for courage I wasn't sure I had. What I wasn't prepared for was how to live after the storm. How to move forward with the same intensity I once reserved for staying alive.

This chapter is my attempt to name what comes next. Not as instruction, but as testimony. Not as closure, but as a continuation of grace.

Because survival isn't the end of a story, it's the beginning of a new one.

A Life Reclaimed, Not Restored

People often imagine a transplant as a restoration, as if the body returns to what it once was. I learned quickly that's not true.

Transplant isn't restoration.
It's a redefinition.

It doesn't erase the years of slow decline, the fatigue, the fear, the resilience. It simply marks a turning point where the body, the mind, and the spirit begin to renegotiate what life can look like on the other side of everything.

I don't feel like the man I was before PKD. I feel like someone forged inside it.

I walk differently.

I think differently.

I pray differently.

I lead differently.

I love differently.

Everything has been sharpened, not softened. Not hardened, either. Sharpened, like someone took the blurry edges of my life and brought them into focus.

The gift of a second chance doesn't make you who you were. It makes you who you were meant to be.

Balancing Gratitude and Grief

Here's something I wish someone had explained years ago:

You can be profoundly grateful for survival and still grieve what it cost.

I grieve the years my family saw me tired.

I grieve the moments fear stole before I knew how to manage it.

I grieve the brother I lost.

I grieve the version of myself who didn't know how limited time could feel.

And yet, intertwined with grief is a gratitude so deep it's difficult to speak aloud.

Gratitude for Ryan.
Gratitude for God's timing.
Gratitude for my wife's steadfast presence.
Gratitude for every student, every colleague, every quiet moment of encouragement.
Gratitude for science, for medicine, for the hands that held mine.
Gratitude for breath, for mornings, for days not promised.

Grief and gratitude are not opposites. They are companions.

The presence of one doesn't diminish the other. They coexist, teaching you how to hold joy with reverence and sorrow with gentleness.

The Future No Longer Feels Borrowed

For nearly two decades, the future felt conditional, like something on loan. Every plan was a "maybe," every dream penciled in lightly, every expectation tentative.

Now, the future feels like something I am allowed to step toward, not with arrogance, but with steadiness.

I no longer ask, *Will I be here in a year?*
Now I ask, *What can I build in the year I've been given?*

There is a difference.

Hope isn't abstract anymore.
It's directional.

I want to teach more.
Write more.
Serve more.
Be present for my family.

Guide my children not only with words, but with example.
Live a faith that is visible in character, not in speeches.

I want to use this borrowed organ and this borrowed grace
wisely.

The Quiet Mission Ahead

Every chapter until now has been about surviving.

This last chapter is about **mission**.

The mission now is simple:

To make my second chance someone else's map.

Not because I have all the answers.
Not because I deserve attention.

But because stories are lanterns, and someone out there is standing in a valley you once walked through.

If my story can give them light, even for a few steps, then I honor the donor who saved me.

I honor the God who carried me.
I honor the people who never left my side.

Sharing the journey doesn't reopen the wounds.
It transforms them into guideposts.

My scars are not signs of damage. They are signs of direction.

What I Know Now

If all the pages of this memoir could be distilled into three truths, they would be these:

1. **You are stronger than the fear that tries to name you.**
   Fear tells you the story is ending. Faith tells you it's changing.

2. **You don't survive alone.** Even when you feel isolated, someone is praying, hoping, standing, or believing on your behalf.

3. **There is always a path forward, especially when you can't yet see it.**

The next step often appears only when you're willing to take it.

Reflection — The Road Beyond the War

When I look back now, I don't see a tragedy.

I don't see a medical file.

I don't see the years lost to scans, labs, or exhaustion.

I see a life reshaped by grace.

A life defined not by disease but by determination.

Not by fear but by faith.

Not by decline but by resilience.

Not by death's shadow but by the stubborn, sacred light that kept showing up in small ways.

A life carried by God, by family, by friends, by medicine, by the quiet courage of ordinary days.

The war is not the whole story.

It was only the valley I walked through to discover the mountain on the other side.

Suppose you're holding this book, whether you are a patient, a caregiver, a student, a leader, a veteran, or simply someone trying to make sense of your own battles. In that case, I hope you hear this clearly:

Your story is not over.

Not yet.

Not now.

Not even close.

There is life beyond the diagnosis.

There is strength beyond the suffering.

There is a purpose beyond the pain.

There is hope beyond the horizon you can currently see.

And sometimes, the quietest wars produce the strongest hearts.

I survived mine.

You can survive yours.

And no matter how dark the valley becomes, you will not walk it alone.

Not then.

Not now.

Not ever.

Using This Appendix

This appendix is designed to help patients, caregivers, and families stay organized, prepared, and engaged throughout the journey with PKD, CKD, transplant evaluation, or chronic illness.

Please Note: These tools are not medical advice; they are simply frameworks that can help you ask questions, track information, and stay involved in your care. Always follow the direction of your medical team.

---

15 Questions to Ask Your Doctor

Practical, empowering, patient-centered questions

Understanding Your Condition

What stage is my kidney disease in, and what does that mean for my daily life?

How quickly has my kidney function changed over time?

Are there symptoms I should monitor more closely?

What tests will I need regularly, and what do they measure?

Medications & Treatment Planning

Are my medications still appropriate for my current kidney function?

What side effects should I expect or look out for?

Is there anything I should avoid (over-the-counter meds, supplements, foods, dehydration, etc.)?

If my condition worsens, what are the next steps in treatment?

Diet, Hydration & Lifestyle

Given my lab values, which nutrients should I be most mindful of: sodium, protein, potassium, phosphorus?

Do you recommend meeting with a renal dietitian?

How much water or fluid intake is appropriate for me right now?

Transplant & Future Planning

When should I begin evaluation for transplant?

Which transplant centers do you recommend and why?

How will we decide the right time to start dialysis, if needed?

Quality of Life & Well-Being

Is there anything else I should be doing to maintain energy, mental health, or daily functioning?

Lab Tracker Sample

Date	Creatinine	eGFR	BUN	Potassium	Hemoglobin	Notes

Diet & Hydration Tracker Sample

Simple, renal-friendly structure — flexible for PKD/CKD

Date	Meals / Notes	Estimated Sodium	Estimated Potassium	Fluid (oz)	How I Felt Today

Fluid Intake & Urine Output Tracker

Date mm/dd/yyyy	Time hh:mm am/pm	Fluid Intake ml	Urine Output ml

Exercise & Activity Tracker

Date	Time hh:mm am/pm	Activity	Minutes Spent 00.00	Estimated Calories	Weight

Helpful Organizations for Patients, Caregivers, Veterans, and Families

The following organizations offer education, support, community, and guidance for individuals navigating chronic illness, kidney disease, transplant preparation, recovery, and the emotional and physical challenges that accompany them. Many also support veterans, caregivers, and families. These resources do **not** replace medical guidance; they serve as trusted places to learn, connect, and receive support.

Kidney, PKD & Transplant Organizations

1. PKD Foundation (PKDCure.org)
The leading nonprofit dedicated to Polycystic Kidney Disease research, education, advocacy, and patient support.

2. National Kidney Foundation (kidney.org)
Provides extensive resources for CKD patients, living donors, transplant recipients, and caregivers.

3. American Association of Kidney Patients (aakp.org)
The largest independent kidney patient organization, offering education, policy advocacy, and patient stories.

4. American Kidney Fund (kidneyfund.org)

Provides financial assistance, education, and prevention programs for kidney patients nationwide.

5. United Network for Organ Sharing (UNOS.org)

Manages the U.S. transplant system and provides donor matching information and patient resources.

6. Donate Life America (donatelife.net)

Focuses on organ donation awareness, registration, and donor family support.

7. Transplant Recipients International Organization (TRIOweb.org)

Offers emotional support, patient mentoring, and community for transplant recipients and families.

8. NephCure Kidney International (nephcure.org)

Supports research and patient education for chronic kidney conditions and rare kidney disorders.

9. Renal Support Network (rsnhope.org)

A patient-led organization offering peer support, education, and community stories.

10. American Society of Transplantation (myAST.org)

Provides transplant-specific education and resources for patients and families.

Chronic Illness, Patient Advocacy & Mental Health

11. Chronic Disease Coalition (chronicdiseasecoalition.org)
Advocates for patient rights and protections for those living with chronic illnesses.

12. Global Genes (globalgenes.org)
Supports people living with rare genetic diseases through resources and community programs.

13. Patient Advocate Foundation (patientadvocate.org)
Offers case management, insurance guidance, and financial navigation services.

14. Mental Health America (mhanational.org)
Provides support, screening tools, and education for emotional well-being during chronic illness.

15. National Alliance on Mental Illness – NAMI (nami.org)
Offers peer groups, education, and support for mental health challenges.

16. Caregiver Action Network (caregiveraction.org)
Support and resources for family caregivers, including educational materials and peer support.

17. The Mighty (themighty.com)

A large online community sharing stories and support for chronic illness and mental health.

18. HealthWell Foundation (healthwellfoundation.org)

Provides financial assistance for medication and treatment costs for chronic disease patients.

Veteran & Military Support Organizations

19. Wounded Warrior Project (woundedwarriorproject.org)

Supports wounded veterans through mental health programs, rehabilitation, and community.

20. Tunnel to Towers Foundation (T2T.org)

Assists families of fallen service members, first responders, and catastrophically injured veterans.

21. USO (uso.org)

Provides support, community, and connection for service members and their families.

22. Team Rubicon (teamrubiconusa.org)

A veteran-led disaster response organization offering purpose and community through service.

23. Disabled American Veterans – DAV (dav.org)

Provides benefits assistance, advocacy, and support services for disabled veterans.

24. Fisher House Foundation (fisherhouse.org)

Provides free lodging near VA and military hospitals for families of hospitalized service members and veterans.

25. Hope for the Warriors (hopeforthewarriors.org)

Supports post-9/11 veterans, service members, and families with health, wellness, and transition programs.

Faith-Based & Inspirational Support

26. Stephen Ministries (stephenministries.org)

Christian caregivers offering one-on-one emotional and spiritual support.

27. GriefShare (griefshare.org)

Faith-informed support groups for individuals experiencing loss or major life changes.

28. Guideposts (guideposts.org)

Provides faith-based stories of hope and resilience for people facing illness and adversity.

Financial, Logistical & Practical Support

29. National Foundation for Transplants (transplants.org)

Helps transplant patients raise funds for medical costs through a structured, transparent platform.

30. The Assistance Fund (tafcares.org)

Offers co-pay and financial assistance programs for individuals with chronic, life-threatening illnesses.

Sources and Further Reading

The following sources informed the medical, biological, and educational context of this memoir. They are provided for readers who wish to deepen their understanding of PKD, chronic kidney disease, transplant preparation, nutrition, patient advocacy, and the science behind kidney function. These resources are *not* intended as medical advice; rather, they offer trusted information, research, and perspectives that may help readers make sense of their own journeys or support someone they love.

Chan, M. et al. (2022). Nutritional management in patients with chronic kidney disease. International Journal of Nephrology, 2022, Article 123456.

Di Lullo, L., et al. (2023). Diet and physical activity in autosomal dominant polycystic kidney disease. Nutrients, 15(11), 2621. https://doi.org/10.3390/nu15112621

Kidney Foundation. (2024). Polycystic kidney disease (PKD): What you need to know. https://www.kidney.org/kidney-topics/polycystic-kidney-disease

Kidney Research UK. (2024). *What do your kidneys do and how do they work?* Retrieved October 10, 2025, from https://www.kidneyresearchuk.org/kidney-health-information/about-kidney-disease/what-the-kidneys-do/ Kidney Research UK

Kim, S. M., & Jung, J. Y. (2020). Nutritional management in patients with chronic kidney disease. Korean Journal of Internal

Medicine, 35(6), 1279–1290.

https://doi.org/10.3904/kjim.2020.408

Mayo Clinic. (n.d.). *Polycystic kidney disease (PKD): Symptoms & causes.*
Retrieved October 10, 2025, from
https://www.mayoclinic.org/diseases-conditions/polycystic-kidney-disease/symptoms-causes/syc-20352820
mayoclinic.org

Mayo Clinic. (2023). *Chronic kidney disease (CKD): Symptoms and causes.*
https://www.mayoclinic.org/diseases-conditions/chronic-kidney-disease/symptoms-causes/syc-20354521

National Institute of Diabetes and Digestive and Kidney Diseases
[NIDDK]. (2023, June 15). Your kidneys & how they work.
https://www.niddk.nih.gov/health-information/kidney-disease/kidneys-how-they-work

National Kidney Foundation [NKF]. (2024). How your kidneys work.
https://www.kidney.org/kidney-topics/how-your-kidneys-work

StatPearls. (2025). Autosomal dominant polycystic kidney disease. In
NCBI Bookshelf. Retrieved October 10, 2025, from
https://www.ncbi.nlm.nih.gov/books/NBK532934/

National Kidney Foundation [NKF]. (2024). How your kidneys work.
https://www.kidney.org/kidney-topics/how-your-kidneys-work

National Kidney Foundation [NKF]. (2024). Potassium in your CKD
diet. https://www.kidney.org/kidney-topics/potassium-your-ckd-diet

National Institute of Diabetes and Digestive and Kidney Diseases (NIDDK). (2024, April 3). *Your kidneys and how they work.* https://www.niddk.nih.gov/health-information/kidney-disease/your-kidneys-how-they-work

NHS. (2024). Autosomal dominant polycystic kidney disease (ADPKD). https://www.nhs.uk/conditions/autosomal-dominant-polycystic-kidney-disease-adpkd/

NIDDK. (2023, May 10). What is polycystic kidney disease (PKD)? U.S. Department of Health and Human Services. https://www.niddk.nih.gov/health-information/kidney-disease/polycystic-kidney-disease/what-is-pkd

Ravindra, T., & others. (2023). Diet and nutrition goals for people with stage 3 chronic kidney disease. DaVita. https://www.davita.com/diet-nutrition/articles/diet-and-nutrition-goals-for-people-with-stage-3-chronic-kidney-disease

Torres, V. E. & Harris, P. C. (2023). Polycystic kidney disease. The New England Journal of Medicine, 389(15), 1361-1372. https://jamanetwork.com/journals/jama/fullarticle/2831904

About the Author

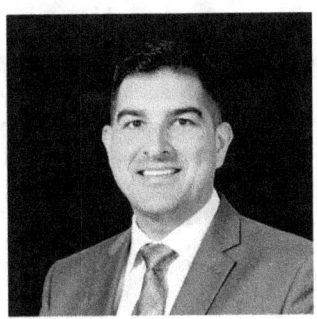

Dr. Daniel O'Connell is a scholar-practitioner, executive leader, and educator whose career bridges digital transformation, governance, and higher education. A U.S. Navy veteran and licensed aviator since 1994, he has flown airplanes, helicopters, and gliders, bringing precision, discipline, and situational awareness to every domain he leads. With over three decades of experience, Dr. O'Connell has led enterprise-scale technology initiatives across sectors, including prior work with RTX (Pratt & Whitney), where he contributed to high-stakes innovation and operational excellence. His expertise spans SAP and Oracle platforms, cybersecurity, and sustainability-aligned governance.

He earned his Doctor of Education (EdD) in 2025, completing his applied research in ethics and use of artificial intelligence in education, and his final manuscript defense in under two years, while serving in a full-time executive role, teaching 3–4 university courses per term, and recovering from a life-saving kidney transplant. His doctoral journey is a testament to resilience, purpose, and the transformative power of education.

Dr. O'Connell teaches in Quinnipiac University's MBA, MSBA, BS Business Analytics, and MS in Cybersecurity programs, where he is known for his governance-aligned instructional design, systems-level thinking, and emotionally accountable mentorship. His prior leadership roles at Yale University and The New School reflect a rare academic pedigree that spans Ivy League, Ivy-adjacent, and regional institutions.

He is the founder and principal of DocLogical, LLC, a premier consulting and advisory firm specializing in AI, Data, Enterprise Systems, Governance, Risk & Compliance (GRC), and Cybersecurity. He also leads DocLogical Press, a publishing imprint dedicated to modular learning, inclusive community scholarship, and cultural heritage, especially within Irish and Celtic traditions.

A proud Connecticut resident for over 30 years, Dr. O'Connell integrates faith-based affirmation, military-informed leadership, and emotionally intelligent communication into every facet of his teaching and service. His mission is to inspire others to dream more, lead with integrity, and build systems that endure.